LIVING WITH

HEART
DISEASE

LIVING WITH

HEART DISEASE

EVERYTHING YOU NEED TO KNOW TO SAFEGUARD YOUR HEALTH AND TAKE CONTROL OF YOUR LIFE

LARRY KATZENSTEIN

ILEANA L. PIÑA, M.D., EDITOR

Professor of Medicine, Case Western Reserve University
Heart Failure Section, Division of Cardiology
Quality Scholar, Louis Stokes VA Medical Center
Cleveland, Ohio

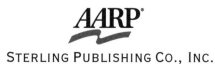

STERLING PUBLISHING CO., INC.

616.12

Kat

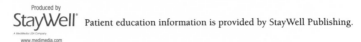
Produced by

StayWell®   Patient education information is provided by StayWell Publishing.

A MediMedia USA Company
www.medimedia.com

AARP Books publishes a wide range of titles on health, personal finance, lifestyle, and other subjects to enrich the lives of older Americans. For more information, please visit www.aarp.org/books.

AARP, established in 1958, is a nonprofit organization with more than 37 million members age 50 or older. The AARP name and logo are registered trademarks of AARP, used under license to Sterling Publishing Co., Inc.

Living with Heart Disease is designed to provide you with health information that can help you become a better-informed, more active consumer of health-care services. It is not intended to be exhaustive on the topic of heart disease, nor does it substitute for the advice of your health-care providers. The science of cardiology is constantly expanding and advancing; the reader is therefore encouraged to check the latest product information, including medication inserts, for potential changes in recommended use. This is especially important when it comes to the use, dosage, or administration of any new or rare drug.

Whereas every attempt has been made to check the content for accuracy, all information is presented without guarantees by the publishers and consultants, who disclaim all liability in connection with its use.

LIBRARY OF CONGRESS CATALOGING-IN-PUBLICATION DATA AVAILABLE

10   9   8   7   6   5   4   3   2   1

Published by Sterling Publishing Co., Inc.
387 Park Avenue South, New York, NY 10016

© 2007 AARP

Distributed in Canada by Sterling Publishing
c/o Canadian Manda Group, 165 Dufferin Street
Toronto, Ontario, Canada M6K 3H6
Distributed in the United Kingdom by GMC Distribution Services
Castle Place, 166 High Street, Lewes, East Sussex, England BN7 1XU
Distributed in Australia by Capricorn Link (Australia) Pty. Ltd.
P.O. Box 704, Windsor, NSW 2756, Australia

Manufactured in the United States of America
All rights reserved

Sterling ISBN-13: 978-1-4027-3011-5
       ISBN-10: 1-4027-3011-X

For information about custom editions, special sales, premium and corporate purchases, please contact Sterling Special Sales Department at 800-805-5489 or specialsales@sterlingpub.com.

Contents

Biographies

Ileana L. Piña, MD, FACC, FAHA

Ileana L. Piña, M.D., received her medical degree from the University of Miami in 1976 and completed a residency in internal medicine at the University of South Florida and a cardiology fellowship at the University of Miami.

Dr. Piña joined the faculty of the University of Miami as Director of the Exercise Laboratory. At the University of Miami, she established the Cardiac Rehabilitation Program and initiated cardiopulmonary testing of heart-failure patients while pursuing a research project using nicorandil in patients with mild to moderate heart failure. In 1987, she joined the faculty at Hahnemann University as Director of Heart Failure and Cardiac Rehabilitation. In 1991, Temple University recruited Dr. Piña to join its Heart Failure Transplant team and to initiate the Cardiac Rehabilitation Program and coordinate the efforts of the Cardiopulmonary Exercise Laboratory. She became the Director of Cardiomyopathy in 1993; was the principal investigator in multiple heart-failure trials including PRECISE (carvedilol), ELITE (losartan), and ATLAS (lisinopril); and served as co-investigator in others such as Bosentan and VEST.

Dr. Piña is Co-Director of the N-HeFt Program, a program that trains cardiologists and primary care physicians in heart failure at Case Western Reserve University with 28 sites in operation nationally. She has written publications in the area of heart failure and has edited two books: *Exercise and Heart Failure* and *The Year in Heart Failure 2004*. Dr. Piña also reviews for *Circulation, American Journal of Cardiology,* and *American Heart Journal*. She sits on the editorial boards of *Journal of Cardiac Rehabilitation* and *Current Cardiology Reports*.

In 1999, Dr. Piña joined the faculty of Case Western Reserve University in Cleveland, Ohio, as Professor of Medicine and Director of the Section of Heart Failure and Cardiac Transplantation in the Department of Medicine, Division of Cardiology at University Hospitals of Cleveland.

Dr. Piña is a past member of the Executive Council and Care Standards Committee of the Heart Failure Society of America. She is Chairperson for the American Heart Association/Heart Failure and Transplantation Committee in the Council on Clinical Cardiology and also serves as an advisor/consultant to the Devices Section of the Food and Drug Administration. A past Chair of the Council on Cardiovascular Rehabilitation and Secondary Prevention of the World Heart Federation, Dr. Piña is as well a past member of the Cardio-Renal Advisory Committee of the Food and Drug Administration.

Faculty Disclosure Statement

Dr. Piña has disclosed that she has received grants from CMS, Biosite; Novartis; and the NIH Institute. She has served on advisory/review panels for AstraZeneca Pharmaceuticals LP and Abbott. She has served as a speaker for AstraZeneca Pharmaceuticals LP; GlaxoSmithKline; Nitromed; and Novartis.

Larry Katzenstein

Larry Katzenstein is a medical writer and editor who relishes making complex subjects comprehensible. He has masters' degrees in biology and journalism. After working for 12 years as a medical writer at *Consumer Reports*, Katzenstein became the medical editor of *American Health Magazine*. Since then, he has written five books, including *Secrets of St. John's Wort; Viagra: The Potency Promise;* and *Taking Charge of Arthritis*.

Katzenstein has written medical articles for a variety of publications, among them *The New York Times, Reader's Digest,* and *Smithsonian Magazine*. He recently served as issue editor for four special editions of *Scientific American* on the topics of ancient art, earth science, physics, and time. Katzenstein is now the science writer for the Albert Einstein College of Medicine in New York City.

Credits

AARP®

Kelly Griffin
SENIOR PROJECT MANAGER
AARP Office of Social Impact
Washington, D.C.

Margaret Hawkins
MANAGER, HEALTH PROMOTION
AARP State & National Initiatives
Washington, D.C.

Keith Lind
SENIOR POLICY ADVISOR
AARP Public Policy Institute
Washington, D.C.

Cheryl Matheis
DIRECTOR, HEALTH STRATEGIES INTEGRATION
AARP Office of Social Impact
Washington, D.C.

N. Lee Rucker
SENIOR POLICY ADVISOR
AARP Public Policy Institute
Washington, D.C.

Illustration Credits

Some illustrations have been adapted from the original content of ▮KRAMES a MediMedia USA company.

Illustrations on pages 41, 94, 95, 96, 97, 98, 99, 100, 101, 102, 103, 109, 136, 143, 152, 157, 207, 210, 225 © 2006 Elliott Golden

Editorial Board

Introduction

Ileana L. Piña, MD

THIS IS A BOOK ABOUT a little-known killer. The killer ranges far and wide, felling more Americans each year than any other cause, and it has done so for nearly two decades now. Despite repeated public-awareness campaigns stressing the dangers it represents, the killer remains at large—largely unrecognized by the American populace, that is.

The killer is heart disease, and according to the American Heart Association more than 70 million Americans—27 million of them age 65 or older—have one or more diseases of the heart or blood vessels (cardiovascular disease). That total includes 65 million people with high blood pressure, 7 million people who have had heart attacks, and another 6 million who suffer angina, or chest pain.

Relentless in its reliability, cardiovascular disease claims another American life every 35 seconds. In 2002, for example, the disease caused 38 percent (912,000) of the nation's 2.4 million total deaths, making it the number one killer in the land. It's a dubious distinction, to be sure—but one that cardiovascular disease has held in the United States since 1900.

In addition to being omnipresent, cardiovascular disease is prompt: According to estimates compiled by the Centers for Disease Control, 400,000 to 460,000 people die each year of heart disease in an emergency department or before they can reach a hospital. That figure represents more than half of all cardiac deaths.

Other statistics shed even more light on the ubiquity of the illness. The chances of having one's first encounter with cardiovascular disease climb steadily with age. By the time you are 85 to 94 years old—two percent of Americans now live that long—your odds of having a run-in with the disease will be eight times higher than they were at 35 to 44. Women typically have their first encounters 10 years later than men. And with the population of the United States aging dramatically—40 million of us will be 65 or older by 2010—it follows that the number of cardiovascular-disease cases will rise commensurately.

Of risk and reward

Not every recent development on the cardiac front has been bleak, however. Thanks to years of painstaking research by cardiologists, nutritionists, and laboratory researchers, the risk factors that predispose a person to develop heart disease—primarily genetics and such lifestyle choices as diet, exercise, and smoking—are now well-known and have been quantified. Knowing what these risks are—and avoiding them, when possible—can save lives.

Many of the risk factors that up the odds of heart disease can be managed. An individual can stop smoking, for example, or take steps to avoid secondhand smoke. He or she can transform a physically inactive existence into an active one, or switch to a diet designed to combat obesity. This last course of action can be especially critical, for high blood pressure, diabetes, and high cholesterol—all common risk factors for heart disease—have soared in lockstep with the "obesity epidemic" in the United States. Whereas only 15 percent of the nation's population was considered obese (more than 30 pounds overweight) in 1966, today that figure has ballooned to a troubling 33 percent. So if you truly want to give your heart a lift, dropping some pounds is a great way to start.

Hope on the horizon

"Knowledge is power," wrote the English author and philosopher Sir Francis Bacon in *Religious Meditations* (1597), and perhaps nowhere does his statement ring truer than in the realm of heart disease prevention and treatment. Here, knowledge alleviates fear of the unknown and its attendant anxiety. Most crucial of all, knowledge saves lives: By identifying your own risk factors early on and taking immediate steps to battle them, you may be able to discourage the development of heart disease.

Those action steps warrant repeating:

- Practice total avoidance of tobacco smoke, be it first- or secondhand.
- Lead as physically active a lifestyle as you can.
- Eat healthy foods.
- Eat in moderation.
- Maintain your ideal weight.

In the event that you are already under a doctor's care for high blood pressure or high cholesterol, take your prescribed medications as directed. Not only can medicines and other treatments developed since the 1970s help ward off heart disease, but they have been shown to improve the survival rate of those with the ailment, allowing countless heart patients to live full and productive lives. Indeed, therapies as yet unperfected may one day succeed in reversing the damage done by heart attacks, returning impaired heart tissue to normal.

Because the odds of developing heart disease rise with age, AARP is committed to informing the public about the ailment's perils and prophylaxis. The accuracy of the information in these pages has been vouchsafed by the medical and health-policy experts profiled on pages x-xi. For additional resources—including what to do in an emergency—see the appendices on pages 251–262.

Where there is education, there is hope. Education fosters self-awareness and with it better self-care, engendering the faith that it is possible to live—indeed, to live well—with heart disease. Bear in mind that the health-care consumer (that is, you, the patient) has an inalienable right to receive complete information about his or her diagnosis and treatment. If this book sparks questions or doubts about your own treatment, by all means voice them. No health care provider should get upset when his or her care is questioned—and should that happen, it's time to shop around for a new doctor.

As a physician who specializes in cardiology, I hope this book will make a positive impact not only on your own life but on the lives of those you love.

The Healthy Heart 1

T HE HEART IS A POWERFUL and durable muscle, but like other body organs it can fall prey to several types of disease. To better understand heart disease and its root causes, you'll need some basic information about this mighty organ and the exceptional job it performs day in and day out. This chapter takes you inside the healthy heart to reveal how it pumps oxygenated (that is, oxygen-rich) blood to wherever it is needed in the human body. As you'll discover, most cases of heart disease in the United States involve clogging of the all-important coronary arteries, which supply blood to the hardworking heart muscle itself.

The Heart Is a Muscle

Small but potent, the heart is about the same size as a balled fist. Clench your fist, relax it, then clench it again. This tightening and relaxing is similar to the way your heart beats. During every minute of your life, the heart contracts and relaxes to pump oxygen-rich blood throughout the body.

This incessant pumping action—squeeze, relax, squeeze, relax—is what creates your heartbeat. When you stop to consider that the normal lifetime heart rate is 60 to 100 beats per minute, you begin to understand why the heart of a 70-year-old person has already beaten more than 2.5 billion times.

The pulse of blood flow created each time the heart contracts is transmitted to your arteries—the vessels that carry blood from the heart to the rest of your body. That's why you can feel your pulse at

1

certain places in your body where large arteries pass just beneath the skin, such as your wrist and neck.

What Your Heart Does

One of the heart's two main jobs is to pump oxygen-rich blood throughout the body. Its other key task is to send this blood to *itself*. Like any other diligent muscle in the body, heart muscle demands a steady supply of oxygenated blood in order to function properly.

Blood vessels called coronary arteries carry oxygenated blood straight into the heart muscle. As this chapter will explain, healthy coronary arteries are crucial to a healthy heart.

Someone whose heart rate is 60 per minute will have more than 86,000 beats each day—and more than two billion in a lifetime.

The coronary arteries are blood vessels that wrap around the surface of the heart. If these essential conduits stay healthy and unclogged, the heart usually gets all the oxygen it needs. It can also quickly increase its oxygen supply when needed, such as during exercise.

If you have heart disease, there is a good chance that part—if not all—of your problem involves diseased (clogged) coronary arteries. The end of this chapter examines how coronary arteries should function in a healthy heart.

Looking inside the Heart

Inside your heart are four chambers (compartments) and four valves. When the heart beats, the valves act like one-way doors. The valves help to regulate the flow of blood as it travels through the heart's chambers and out to the lungs and body.

The interior of the heart is divided into right and left sides. Each side has an upper chamber called an atrium and a lower chamber called a ventricle. The two upper chambers (atria) receive

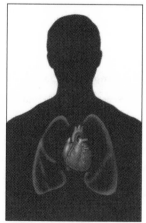

> The heart is located between the lungs, near the center of the chest.

- **Aorta:** the large artery that carries blood from the heart to the rest of the body.
- **Artery:** one of the branching vessels or tubes that carry blood from the heart to various parts of the body.
- **Atria:** the heart's two upper chambers; they receive blood from the rest of the body or from the lungs.
- **AV (atrioventricular) node:** a bundle of cells that send electrical signals into the ventricles.
- **Coronary arteries:** blood vessels that wrap around the heart and supply the heart muscle with blood.
- **Myocardium:** heart muscle.
- **Pulmonary artery:** the large blood vessel that carries blood from the heart to the lungs.
- **Sinoatrial (SA) node:** a bundle of electrical cells that set the pace of the heartbeat; sometimes called the heart's pacemaker.
- **Valve:** a membranous flap that opens and closes to let blood flow from one chamber of the heart to another.
- **Vein:** one of the branching vessels or tubes that convey blood from various parts of the body to the heart.
- **Ventricles:** the heart's two lower chambers; they pump blood to the body and lungs.

blood from the lungs or the body. When the atria contract, they pump blood into the two ventricles beneath them. As the ventricles contract, they pump blood to the lungs or the body.

Your heart is your strongest muscle. Each day it pumps about 2,100 gallons of blood.

A Fantastic Voyage through the Heart

To better understand how blood travels through the heart and out to the body, consider just one of its four chambers: the right atrium. This chamber receives "used" blood—that is to say, blood that has already flowed through the body, giving up its oxygen along the way

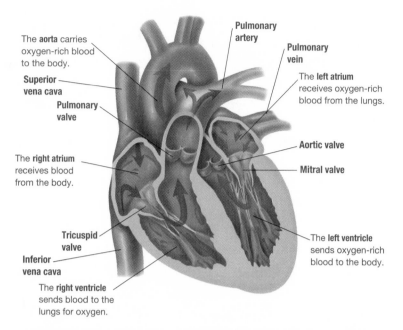

The **aorta** carries oxygen-rich blood to the body.

Superior vena cava

Pulmonary valve

The **right atrium** receives blood from the body.

Tricuspid valve

Inferior vena cava

The **right ventricle** sends blood to the lungs for oxygen.

Pulmonary artery

Pulmonary vein

The **left atrium** receives oxygen-rich blood from the lungs.

Aortic valve

Mitral valve

The **left ventricle** sends oxygen-rich blood to the body.

> The heart is a lovely pumper. Each chamber, valve, and tube in the human heart serves a special purpose, yet all must act in syncopation to keep blood—and therefore oxygen—flowing freely to the body's various tissues.

to the cells of muscles, organs, and other tissues that need it. After being collected from these tissues by veins all over the body, the used blood is funneled into the right atrium through two extra-large veins, the superior vena cava (which carries blood from your head and arms) and the inferior vena cava (which carries blood from your legs and abdomen).

Blood in the veins (venous blood) is a dark bluish-red color because its oxygen content is used up. By contrast, the oxygen in arterial blood gives it a bright-red color.

When the right atrium contracts, it sends oxygen-depleted blood down into the right ventricle. The right ventricle then contracts in turn, pumping the used blood through the pulmonary artery to the lungs, which restore the blood's oxygen level. This freshly oxygenated blood flows from the lungs into the pulmonary vein and then back to the heart, where it enters the left atrium.

In the last step of its journey through the heart, the oxygen-rich blood in the left atrium is pumped into perhaps the most important of the heart's four chambers, the muscular left ventricle. As shown on the facing page, the left ventricle's walls are the thickest of all four chambers. The left ventricle needs this extra muscle power to propel the oxygen-rich blood out of the heart with enough force for it to reach every part of the body.

Each atrium is about the size of a golf ball.

The left ventricle pumps this blood through an extra-large artery called the aorta, which branches into smaller arteries that deliver oxygen-rich blood to the rest of the body. Once the body has used up the oxygen, veins return the spent blood to the right atrium and the cycle begins anew.

As the illustration below makes clear, not all of the oxygen-rich blood pumped through the aorta travels to the rest of the body; some is sent via the coronary arteries to nourish the heart itself.

Keeping the Beat

The heart has a natural pacemaker—the sinoatrial (SA) node—that ensures the heart pumps blood in a steady rhythm. At regular intervals, the SA node (consisting of a bundle of specialized cells in the right atrium) emits electrical signals that spread throughout the heart

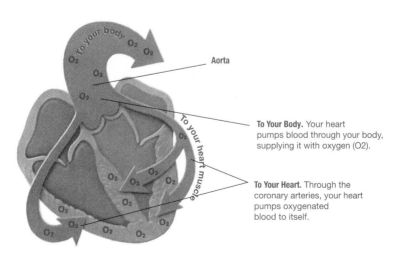

Aorta

To Your Body. Your heart pumps blood through your body, supplying it with oxygen (O2).

To Your Heart. Through the coronary arteries, your heart pumps oxygenated blood to itself.

> Most of the oxygen-rich blood pumped from your heart goes out to your body via the aorta, supplying tissues from head to toe with the oxygen they need to stay alive and function efficiently. But some of this blood goes through the coronary arteries right back into the heart itself, providing heart muscle with the oxygen it needs.

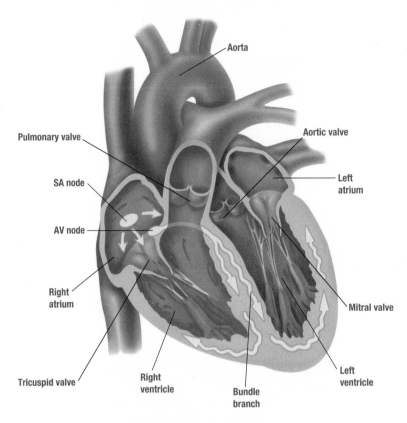

Aorta

Pulmonary valve

Aortic valve

SA node

Left
atrium

AV node

Right
atrium

Mitral valve

Tricuspid valve

Right
ventricle

Bundle
branch

Left
ventricle

> Groups of special cells in the right atrium, called nodes, send the heart's electrical
signals. The signals originate in the sinoatrial (SA) node and travel along pathways.
In the ventricles, these pathways are called bundle branches. The atrioventricular
(AV) node sends electrical signals into the ventricles.

muscle and trigger each chamber of the heart to pump in sequence.
First, the electrical signals tell the atria to squeeze, opening the mitral and tricuspid valves and forcing blood into the ventricles. Next,
the electrical signals tell the ventricles to squeeze, opening the aortic
and pulmonary valves and sending blood to the body and lungs.

Coronary Arteries Are Key

The majority of heart-disease cases involve the coronary arteries—
those vessels visible on the heart's surface that supply the hardworking heart muscle with oxygen-rich blood. Coronary arteries
therefore play a vital role in heart health.

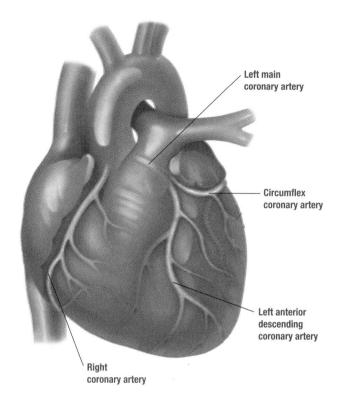

Left main coronary artery

Circumflex coronary artery

Left anterior descending coronary artery

Right coronary artery

> When the heart is viewed from the outside, some blood vessels are visible on its surface. These are the coronary arteries. They are blood vessels that wrap around the surface of the heart and supply the heart muscle beneath with oxygen-rich blood.

The coronary arteries branch off the aorta (the largest artery that leaves the heart). These spread out over the surface of the heart to supply it oxygenated blood. The left main coronary artery splits into two branches—the circumflex and left anterior—and furnishes oxygen-rich blood to the front, left side, and top of the heart muscle. The right coronary artery provides oxygen-rich blood to the back, right side, and bottom of the heart muscle.

> Each ventricle holds approximately 1/8 of a cup of blood after it contracts and about 1/2 cup once it refills.

Examining the coronary arteries from the outside cannot reveal how healthy they are. Only by looking inside the arteries can one see whether they are wide enough and flexible enough to carry all the blood your heart needs.

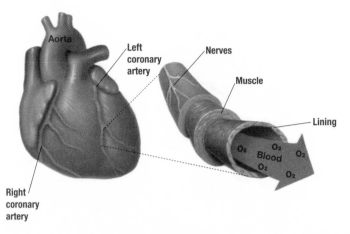

> Healthy coronary arteries are elastic and have smooth interior linings, allowing blood to flow freely. Like all arteries, the ones supplying the heart have muscles that contract and relax in response to signals from surrounding nerves, letting more or less blood flow to the heart.

So great is the heart muscle's thirst for oxygen that it uses nearly all the oxygen that passes through it. When the coronary arteries are healthy, they allow the heart to quickly boost its oxygen supply as needed—during periods of exercise, for example.

Blood flows freely through coronary arteries with smooth linings, allowing the proper amount of oxygen to reach the heart muscle. The coronary arteries widen to meet the heart's increased demand. This allows them to carry more blood—and thus deliver more oxygen to the heart muscle.

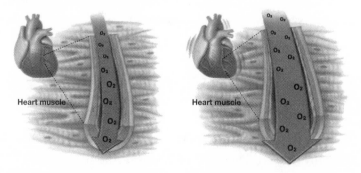

> Coronary arteries widen with physical activity to supply the heart with the oxygenated blood it requires.

The coronary arteries' ability to supply heart muscle with oxygen-rich blood is of critical importance to the health of your heart. As detailed in Chapter 4, diagnostic tests such as a stress test can gauge the health of your coronary arteries.

When you're resting

As you sit quietly reading this book, your heart keeps working. Each minute, it beats 60 to 80 times and pumps more than a gallon of blood throughout your body. In order to maintain this steady state of intensity, your heart demands a steady supply of oxygen. You feel comfortable because your heart's oxygen supply equals its demand.

When you're active

When you become more active, so does your heart. It almost doubles its speed and pumps more blood each minute to fuel your body's work. Because it is pumping faster, your heart also demands more oxygen. You continue to feel comfortable because your heart is still getting the oxygen it demands.

During strenuous exercise, your heart may pump four to seven times as much blood as it does when you're at rest.

What Is Heart Disease? 2

T HE HEART IS A COMPLEX ORGAN. Its diverse structures perform a rich array of unique functions, so it's no surprise that
"heart disease" is not a single illness but a catchall term encompass-
ing several different ailments. One of those conditions—coronary
artery disease, or CAD—is the most common type of heart disease.
Indeed, CAD exceeds cancer as the No. 1 cause of death in the
United States. Other types of heart disease can undermine the organ's rhythm and pumping power, its valves and arteries, and the
heart muscle itself.

This chapter describes the various diseases that can affect the
heart. It also discusses other health problems, such as stroke, that
are caused by the same underlying artery damage responsible for
most cases of heart disease.

One common heart problem is atrial fibrillation, in which the upper chambers of the heart beat very quickly and unevenly. Other heart
diseases include heart-valve disease (when the heart's valves don't open
or close as they should) and problems of the heart mus-
cle itself, which are commonly known as cardiomyopathies. Heart failure, in which the heart muscle becomes weaker and unable to pump with enough force,
is the most common discharge diagnosis—that is, the
reason for a hospital stay after a hospital assessment—for patients over
65. Heart failure can result from coronary artery disease, diseases of the
valves, or cardiomyopathies. It is the only form of heart disease whose
incidence continues to rise among the U.S. population.

> Coronary artery disease is the single largest killer of American men and women.

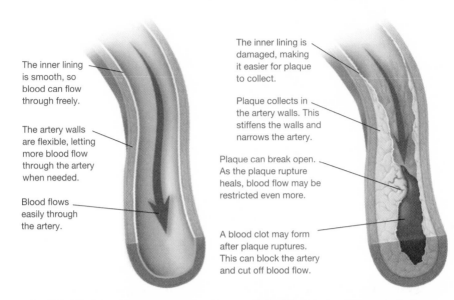

The inner lining is smooth, so blood can flow through freely.

The artery walls are flexible, letting more blood flow through the artery when needed.

Blood flows easily through the artery.

The inner lining is damaged, making it easier for plaque to collect.

Plaque collects in the artery walls. This stiffens the walls and narrows the artery.

Plaque can break open. As the plaque rupture heals, blood flow may be restricted even more.

A blood clot may form after plaque ruptures. This can block the artery and cut off blood flow.

> **Healthy Arteries.** Arteries are blood vessels that carry oxygen-rich blood. Healthy arteries have flexible walls and smooth inner linings. Because the arteries are flexible and smooth, blood flows freely through them to deliver oxygen all over the body.

> **Unhealthy Arteries.** Damage to the inner lining of a coronary artery lets cholesterol and other harmful lipids (fats in the blood) gather on the inner artery wall to form fatty deposits, or plaque. This thickens the artery wall and constricts its channel.

The ABCs of Coronary Artery Disease

As described in chapter 1, coronary arteries are crucial blood vessels that supply blood to the heart muscle itself. In coronary artery disease (CAD), the channel, or opening, inside the coronary arteries becomes narrowed or blocked, restricting the flow of oxygen-rich blood to the heart muscle.

CAD starts when the inner lining of a coronary artery is damaged. This is often due to a risk factor, such as smoking or high blood cholesterol. (The risk factors for CAD are discussed in more detail in the next chapter.)

If the inner lining of a coronary artery is damaged, cholesterol and other harmful lipids (fats in the blood) as well as calcium and scar tissue can accumulate within the artery wall to form a gunky material called plaque. As plaque builds up, it thickens the artery wall and narrows its channel, so that not as much blood can flow through.

The accumulation of these fat-laden plaque deposits—a disease process known as atherosclerosis—is fueled by inflammation within the artery wall.

A tough, scar-like "cap" usually forms over the fatty core of a plaque, which helps to safely wall the plaque off from the blood. Scientists now believe that most heart attacks—as well as many strokes—occur when a plaque deposit's fibrous cap ruptures, allowing the plaque's contents to spill into the blood. Blood clots that form over these ruptured plaques may then block the artery, leading to heart attacks and strokes.

What Is a Heart Attack?

A heart attack occurs when part of the heart muscle beyond the coronary-artery blockage receives no oxygen and, as a result, is permanently damaged. The longer the heart muscle is deprived of oxygen, the more extensive the damage. This is why early intervention—to remove the clot, restore blood flow, and minimize heart-muscle damage—is crucially important when a heart attack occurs.

The Warning Signs of Angina

Nearly half of all fatal heart attacks befall individuals who have never shown symptoms of CAD. But some people are luckier: Before artery clogging from CAD becomes severe enough to cause a heart attack, the decreased blood flow may bring on the symptoms of heart disease known as angina (decreased oxygen to the heart).

This year, an estimated 1.2 million Americans will have a heart attack—700,000 will have a first heart attack, and 500,000 will have a repeat one.

Angina is often described as "chest pain," but that label can be misleading. Angina is not always painful, nor is it always felt in the chest. In fact, the symptoms of angina can vary from person to person, and women often experience different symptoms from men. The one constant is each person's angina symptoms: Your symptoms will most likely remain the same from one attack to the next, although they may increase in frequency or intensity.

This is how angina might feel:

- You may have pain, heaviness, tightness, pressure, burning, aching, or feelings of indigestion.
- These sensations may emanate from the chest, back, neck, throat, or jaw. Angina may also be felt in the arms, elbows, wrists, or shoulders.
- Other symptoms may occur at the same time. These include tiredness, nausea and vomiting, sweating, shortness of breath, lightheadedness, increased heart rate, or irregular heart rate.
- In some cases, notably in those with diabetes, a person's decreased sensation may keep angina symptoms from surfacing.

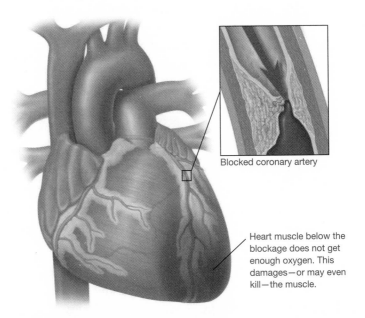

Blocked coronary artery

Heart muscle below the blockage does not get enough oxygen. This damages—or may even kill—the muscle.

> **Your Heart May Be at Risk**

Plaque and blood clots in coronary arteries can interrupt blood flow to the heart when:

- a coronary artery narrows, reducing blood flow to the heart—and often leading to symptoms of angina.
- a coronary artery gets blocked, stopping blood flow beyond the blockage. The resulting lack of oxygen often damages the muscle. If the muscle goes without oxygen for too long, the deprived part of the heart muscle dies.

Thus—and somewhat paradoxically—a heart-disease patient may experience less angina as he or she grows older.

• Women frequently feel neck, shoulder, or mid-back pain, nausea, indigestion, fatigue, dizziness, palpitations, and shortness of breath.

Angina is not the same as a heart attack. The crucial distinction is that angina does not cause lasting damage to the heart. It is, however, a symptom of heart disease—a signal that you have an elevated risk of suffering a heart attack. Fortunately, several steps are available to relieve your symptoms and decrease that risk.

The Two Types of Angina

There are two kinds of angina: stable and unstable. Both types need to be treated. If you have had angina for less than six months, it may be treated as unstable until it is shown to be stable. Call your doctor right away if your angina begins to occur more often, lasts longer, occurs at rest, or causes more discomfort.

Stable angina occurs at predictable times—when you're doing something active, for example, such as climbing stairs. It may also be triggered by anger or stress. Stable angina does not occur during rest. In fact, rest relieves symptoms within a few minutes.

Unstable angina—a sign that a heart attack is likely in the near future—is not predictable. It can occur during rest, and its attacks last longer than they typically do with stable angina.

CAD by itself is clearly a serious disease, given that it raises your risk of suffering a heart attack. But CAD is implicated in several other forms of heart disease as well. It can cause heart failure, cardiomyopathy, and certain types of heart-valve disease.

About 20 percent of heart attack victims have had angina for quite some time.

CAD can also reach beyond the heart to other parts of the body. That's because atherosclerosis—the disease process that causes CAD by clogging coronary arteries—can harm arteries *outside* the heart, too.

For example, arteries in the brain that are affected by atherosclerosis are vulnerable to blood clots that result in strokes. And when atherosclerosis besets arteries in the legs, the result can be aches and cramping. In addition, the kidneys and the aorta (the body's main artery) can become clogged and narrowed.

If you've been diagnosed with CAD, you can take action to keep it from getting worse and to keep it from causing a heart attack. And if you've already experienced a heart attack, you can help prevent CAD from causing another one. As a bonus, your efforts in treating CAD—adopting a low-fat diet, exercising, quitting tobacco, or taking drugs to lower the cholesterol in your blood—can keep arteries from clogging in other parts of your body.

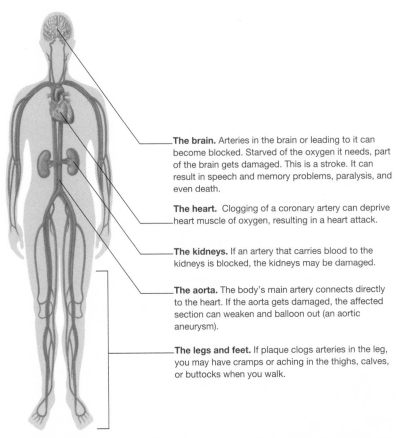

The brain. Arteries in the brain or leading to it can become blocked. Starved of the oxygen it needs, part of the brain gets damaged. This is a stroke. It can result in speech and memory problems, paralysis, and even death.

The heart. Clogging of a coronary artery can deprive heart muscle of oxygen, resulting in a heart attack.

The kidneys. If an artery that carries blood to the kidneys is blocked, the kidneys may be damaged.

The aorta. The body's main artery connects directly to the heart. If the aorta gets damaged, the affected section can weaken and balloon out (an aortic aneurysm).

The legs and feet. If plaque clogs arteries in the leg, you may have cramps or aching in the thighs, calves, or buttocks when you walk.

> **Bottlenecks in the Body.** Plaque can build up and rupture in arteries anywhere in the body, causing the problems listed above.

Cardiomyopathy

Those with cardiomyopathy—heart-muscle disease—have a problem with the muscle tissue that makes up the heart. This means the heart may not be pumping as well as it should.

Cardiomyopathy is not an uncommon condition. Of the three types of cardiomyopathy—dilated, hypertrophic, and restrictive—only the first occurs with any degree of prevalence.

Symptoms of Dilated Cardiomyopathy

Dilated cardiomyopathy often causes no symptoms. If symptoms do occur, they often happen when you exert yourself. Symptoms may include:

- Problems catching your breath
- Unexplained tiredness
- Lightheadedness, dizzy spells, or fainting
- Rapid, pounding heartbeat
- Chest tightness or pressure
- Fluid retention resulting in swollen feet or ankles or unexplained weight gain

Cardiomyopathy doesn't go away, but drugs (or possibly even surgery) can be used to treat it. Such treatment can help keep cardiomyopathy from getting worse and can reduce your symptoms. In addition, treatment of cardiomyopathy can help prevent heart failure.

Heart Failure

When you have heart failure, your heart can't move as much blood as it should with each beat. Certain organs therefore do not receive enough blood to function normally, causing the symptoms you feel.

In most cases, heart failure is caused by another health problem—often by a heart attack but also by high blood pressure or heart-valve disease.

Here are some of the most common heart-failure symptoms. You may have many of these or only a few.

- Shortness of breath, wheezing, or coughing when you exert yourself
- Weakness or tiredness after little effort
- Problems breathing when you're lying flat or the need to sleep in a recliner or propped up on many pillows
- Waking up at night coughing or short of breath
- Rapid weight gain
- Swelling in the abdomen, ankles, or feet
- Cough that could be confused with bronchitis or the common cold
- Abdominal symptoms such as feeling full early, bloating, and loss of appetite

Heart failure can happen in two ways. You may have one or both types.

With systolic dysfunction, the heart muscle becomes weak and enlarged. The weakened muscle doesn't pump enough blood forward when the ventricles contract.

Nearly five million Americans are living with heart failure; 550,000 new cases are diagnosed each year.

With diastolic dysfunction, the heart muscle becomes stiff and thick. The stiff muscle can't fully relax between contractions, preventing the ventricles from filling with enough blood.

When the heart cannot pump enough blood, body chemicals known as hormones are sent out to make the heart work harder. Some of these hormones cause the heart muscle to grow larger. Others instruct the heart to pump faster. This may help move blood at first, but the heart muscle can't keep pace with the demands. Over time, the extra work damages the heart even further.

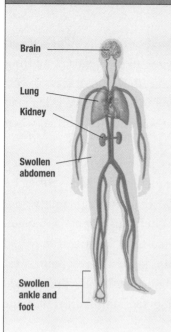

Brain

Lung

Kidney

Swollen
abdomen

Swollen
ankle and
foot

Because a weakened heart muscle moves less blood with each pump, fluid backs up into the lungs and throughout the body. This causes swelling. Less blood moving through your body also means your organs get less oxygen, preventing them from functioning well. This may result in symptoms all over your body:

- Your brain may receive less blood, making you feel confused or dizzy.
- Your lungs may fill with fluid, leaving you short of breath.
- Your kidneys may not be able to rid your body of excess fluid. This fluid can back up into other parts of your body.
- Your abdomen, ankles, and feet may collect excess fluid, causing swelling.

Peripheral Arterial Disease (PAD)

PAD occurs when arteries in the legs become constricted and blocked. This interferes with blood flow to the legs and feet. Though there is no known cure for PAD, you can reduce the cramping and other symptoms of PAD—and slow the progress of the disease—by changing certain aspects of your lifestyle, such as exercising more and stopping smoking.

PAD can cause cramping or aching in your buttocks, thighs, or calves after a short walk. This pain, called claudication, goes away when you stop, but it returns when you move again. The claudication is likely to be more intense when you climb stairs or walk up-hill. As PAD worsens you may have pain more often.

The artery clogging of PAD is caused by atherosclerosis, the same disease process that narrows coronary arteries in CAD. And PAD is initiated by the same risk factors (cigarette smoking and high blood-cholesterol levels, for example) implicated in CAD. This means that PAD is a warning that arteries elsewhere in your body may also be narrowed.

In PAD, leg arteries that are narrowed but not yet blocked can usually provide enough blood and oxygen to your muscles during rest. But when you're active, they cannot meet the increased demand for blood. As a result, your leg may ache or cramp when you walk but feel normal when you are sitting still.

> Cigarette smoking is a big risk factor for PAD, which affects about eight million Americans—including 12 to 20 percent of those 65 and older.

In cases of severe peripheral artery disease, a leg artery can become completely blocked—either by plaque or by a blood clot that lodges in a narrowed section of the artery. When this happens, oxygen cannot reach the muscle below the blockage. Then you may feel pain when lying down. This type of pain, known as rest pain, is especially common at night when you're lying flat. In time the affected tissue can die, sometimes necessitating the amputation of a toe or foot.

Heart-Valve Disease

Heart valves are doorways that keep blood flowing through the chambers of the heart in a single direction. They open and close as blood moves through them, with each valve in the heart opening and closing once with each heartbeat. Having heart-valve disease means that something is keeping one or more of these valves from opening or closing properly. Though valve disease may sometimes be serious, it often responds to treatment.

Rheumatic fever, typically a childhood infection, was once the most common cause of heart-valve problems. Today, by contrast, rheumatic fever has become rare, and valve disease is more often caused by calcium deposits that accumulate on valves as people age. In addition, some people may be born with a problem valve or a tendency to develop problem valves. Coronary artery disease, with its frequent result of blocked blood vessels in the heart, can occasionally precipitate certain types of heart-valve disease. Alternatively, a heart infection may damage one or more valves.

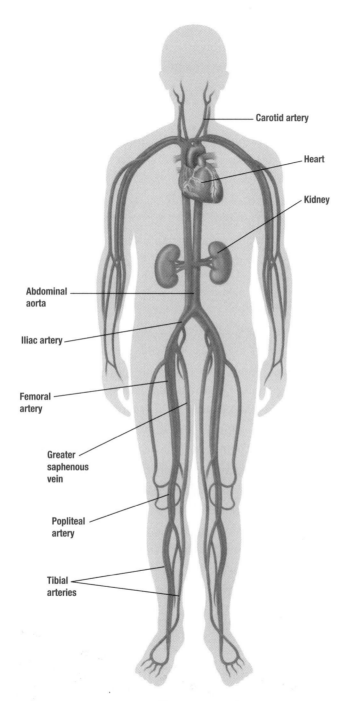

Carotid artery

Heart

Kidney

Abdominal
aorta

Iliac artery

Femoral
artery

Greater
saphenous
vein

Popliteal
artery

Tibial
arteries

> With peripheral artery disease (PAD), a leg can have more than one blockage.

Symptoms of Heart-Valve Disease

Heart-valve problems frequently trigger no symptoms at all. If you do feel symptoms, they may include:

- Wheezing, coughing, or shortness of breath when you exert yourself
- Problems breathing when lying down; waking up at night coughing or feeling short of breath
- Swollen ankles or feet
- Weakness or tiredness
- Chest pain or pressure
- Fast, pounding heartbeat or a fluttering feeling in your chest
- Dizzy spells; fainting spells

Types of Heart-Valve Problems

Valve disease occurs when a valve does not open or close the way it was designed to. If a valve opens only partway, for example, the heart must push blood through a smaller opening. If the valve does not close tight, some blood will leak backward. In either case, the heart may have to work harder to move the same amount of blood. In time, this extra work may tire and weaken the heart muscle.

The telltale heart may not exist outside an Edgar Allan Poe story, but the telltale valve certainly does. A heart valve that is not functioning properly will usually emit a distinctive noise. A stethoscope can detect this noise, called a heart murmur. Be aware, however, that the mere presence of a heart murmur does not mean you have valve disease—or any other heart problem, for that matter. It may simply indicate that your heart beats in an irregular harmless rhythm. Diagnostic tests such as echocardiography can confirm or refute the suspected existence of valve disease.

Any valve in the heart can develop a problem, but the aortic and mitral valves are the ones most commonly afflicted. Tricuspid-valve problems are less common. Pulmonic-valve problems, also rare, are almost always present from birth, but only rarely can they be diagnosed before adulthood.

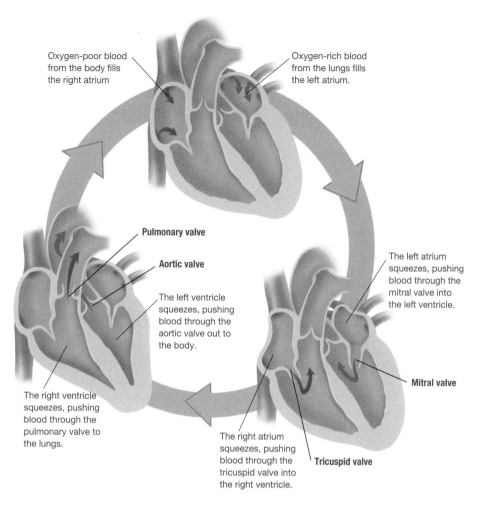

Oxygen-poor blood from the body fills the right atrium

Oxygen-rich blood from the lungs fills the left atrium.

Pulmonary valve

Aortic valve

The left ventricle squeezes, pushing blood through the aortic valve out to the body.

The left atrium squeezes, pushing blood through the mitral valve into the left ventricle.

Mitral valve

The right ventricle squeezes, pushing blood through the pulmonary valve to the lungs.

The right atrium squeezes, pushing blood through the tricuspid valve into the right ventricle.

Tricuspid valve

> The four heart valves work in concert to move blood efficiently through the organ. With each contraction of the heart muscle, the valves open and close to keep blood moving forward.

Problems Affecting the Aortic Valve

Aortic stenosis

A diagnosis of aortic stenosis means your aortic valve has difficulty opening. As a result, the left ventricle has to work harder to push the blood through the valve and out to the body. In some cases, this extra work will make the muscle of the ventricle thicken. With the passage of time, the extra work can tire the heart and cause the heart muscle to weaken. This type of stenosis can quickly get worse.

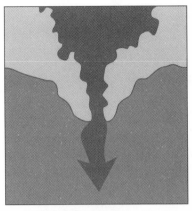

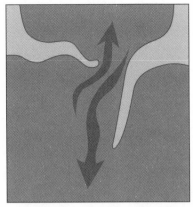

> **Problems Opening (Stenosis).**
When a valve doesn't open all the way,
the problem is called stenosis.
Scarring or deposits of calcium may
make the valve stiff and hard to open.
The resulting narrowed channel forces
blood to flow through a smaller
opening—which, in turn, requires the
heart muscle to work harder to push
the blood through. Stenosis can get
worse over time.

> **Problems Closing (Insufficiency).**
When the valve doesn't close tight,
the problem is called insufficiency
(or regurgitation). The valve may
have extra tissue, it may be loose or
shortened, or the structures support-
ing it may be torn. A valve that doesn't
seal completely lets blood leak
backward through the valve. The heart
must then move some of the same
blood again.

Aortic stenosis may result
from calcium deposits that can
form on the aortic valve as you get
older. These deposits make the
valve stiff and hard to open. In
some cases, you may have been
born with a problematic aortic
valve. Or your aortic valve may
have been damaged by rheumatic
fever.

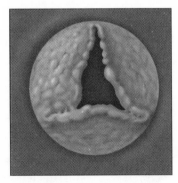

> Open aortic valve with stenosis
(viewed from above).

In many cases, treatment for
aortic stenosis is not needed unless you have symptoms. If you do
have symptoms, medications may help relieve them. If the stenosis
is severe, your doctor may recommend surgery to replace the valve.

Aortic insufficiency

Aortic insufficiency (a condition also known as aortic regurgitation or aortic incompetence) means the aortic valve has problems closing. As a result, blood leaks back through the valve. This extra blood may cause the ventricle to stretch. A stretched ventricle cannot do its main job—that is, to squeeze—as well as it should. As a result, over

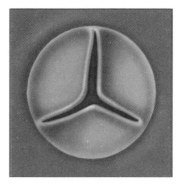

> Closed aortic valve with insufficiency (viewed from above).

time the heart loses its ability to move blood the way it's supposed to. If you have aortic insufficiency, you may have been born with the problem. Alternatively, rheumatic fever or a heart infection may have damaged your aortic valve.

Aortic insufficiency can be treated with prescription drugs that ease the heart's pumping burden. One such therapy is the drug class known as diuretics; these rid the body of excess fluid, giving the heart that much less blood to pump. Another drug class, beta blockers, lighten the cardiac load by slowing the heart rate. Drugs may not suffice to treat severe insufficiency, however; in that case heart-valve surgery may be required, especially if you develop symptoms.

Mitral-valve prolapse

"Prolapse" means the falling down of an organ or other part of the body from its normal position. In mitral-valve prolapse—the most common heart-valve problem—the valve bulges slightly back into the atrium when it closes, allowing a tiny amount of blood to leak. Minor symptoms such as mild chest pain or palpitations may occur.

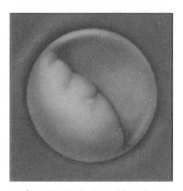

> Closed mitral valve with prolapse (viewed from above).

Mitral-valve prolapse is usually not serious. In some cases, though, it can progress to serious mitral insufficiency.

Mitral-valve prolapse is often present from birth. Simple wear and tear or other, more complex health problems may also cause the condition to emerge later in life. Your tendency to have it may be inherited. For reasons that medical researchers have yet to unlock, mitral-valve prolapse is more common in women than in men.

Unless its symptoms are severe, mitral-valve prolapse rarely needs treatment. Medications can help relieve bothersome symptoms such as anxiety that afflict many people with this disorder. Your doctor may ask you to come in from time to time for tests to check your heart valve and to make sure the problem is not worsening.

Mitral insufficiency

This condition means that your mitral valve has problems closing, letting blood leak back through the valve. Mild cases of mitral insufficiency—those in which only a small amount of blood leaks—rarely cause problems. Severe cases, by contrast, can eventually harm the ventricle and heart muscle.

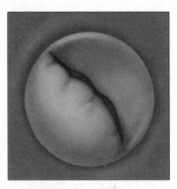

> Closed mitral valve with insufficiency (viewed from above).

Heart damage stemming from a disease such as rheumatic fever may cause mitral insufficiency. Aging, pure and simple, can also bring it on. In some cases, mitral insufficiency may result from mitral-valve prolapse.

More serious cases of mitral insufficiency may necessitate the use of medications to help the heart work more efficiently. In severe cases, heart-valve surgery may be required to repair or replace the valve.

Mitral stenosis

In mitral stenosis, the mitral valve stiffens and cannot open properly. Blood must move through a smaller opening. In severe cases, fluid can build up in the lungs, leading to breathing problems and coughing. Problems with the mitral valve can also trigger a fast or irregular heartbeat (palpitations). Mitral stenosis may slowly get worse over time.

Most cases of mitral stenosis are caused by rheumatic fever in childhood, which can lead to an inflammation that damages the heart valves. Though pregnancy is not responsible for the condition, a woman may first develop symptoms during pregnancy. The reason: The amount of blood her heart must move has increased.

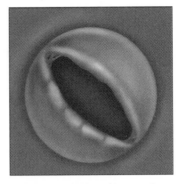

> Open mitral valve with stenosis (viewed from above).

If mitral stenosis is causing no symptoms, then no treatment is usually required. If symptoms occur, on the other hand, your doctor may prescribe medications to ease them. And if the stenosis is severe, surgery can repair or replace the valve.

Atrial Fibrillation

Atrial fibrillation is an arrhythmia (a disturbance in the rhythm of the heartbeat) that causes the heart to beat too fast. Also called "atrial fib" or "A-fib," this common heart problem involves the atria, the upper two chambers of the heart.

Atrial fibrillation can result in annoying symptoms. Though rarely life-threatening, A-fib can lead to serious health problems such as stroke or heart failure. Fortunately, these problems can often be prevented by careful management of the arrhythmia.

How you might feel

If you have atrial fibrillation, you may have experienced one or more of the following:

- Palpitations (fluttering, fast heartbeat)
- Weakness or tiredness
- Shortness of breath
- Chest pain or tightness
- Dizziness or lightheadedness
- Fainting spells

Defects in the heart's electrical system make the atria beat faster than normal. If the atria beat quickly but evenly, the problem is called atrial flutter. If the atria beat unevenly and very quickly, the condition is dubbed atrial fibrillation. In either case, the atria may beat quickly only once in a while (paroxysmal), or they may beat quickly all the time (chronic). Atrial flutter or atrial fibrillation can be prompted by a range of factors—heart attack, high blood pressure, a thyroid problem—or they may have no known cause at all.

Flutter and Fibrillation: What's the Diff?

In atrial flutter, electrical signals travel around and around inside the atria. These circling signals tell the atria to beat quickly (around 200 to 300 beats per minute, or bpm). Some of the signals make it through the atrioventricular node to the ventricles, instructing those lower chambers to beat quickly too (up to 150 bpm).

Atrial flutter can cause symptoms similar to those of atrial fibrillation. It can also lead to the even faster, uneven rhythms of atrial fibrillation.

With atrial fibrillation, cells in the atria emit extra electrical signals. These extra signals make the atria beat not only very quickly (from 400 to 500 bpm) but also unevenly. (The ventricles, for their part, may beat as fast as 180 bpm.) Indeed, the atria beat so fast and so unevenly that they may quiver rather than contract.

If the atria do not contract, they cannot move enough blood into the ventricles. This brings on symptoms such as dizziness and weakness. Worst of all, blood that is not kept moving can pool—and then form clots—in the atria. These clots can move into other parts of the body and cause serious problems, such as a stroke.

The Risk of Stroke

Plaque can narrow arteries anywhere in the body—not just those in the heart. One of the most dangerous places for this to occur is in the arteries of the brain. Just as stanching the flow of blood to heart muscle can precipitate a heart attack, obstructing blood flow in the

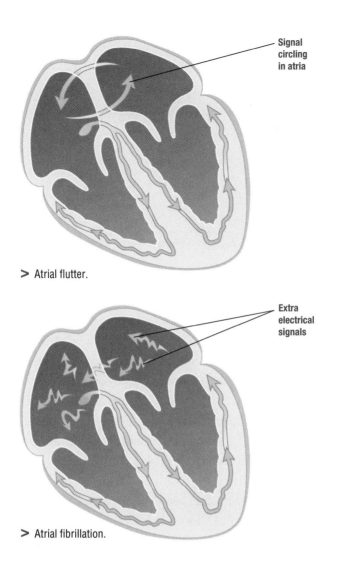

> Atrial flutter.

> Atrial fibrillation.

brain can cause a stroke. In fact, stroke is sometimes referred to as "brain attack."

Like the heart, the brain depends on arteries for its supply of oxygen-rich blood. By the same token, the process of plaque buildup that causes CAD (the most common type of heart disease) can also narrow or block cerebral arteries. Not only that, but leakage or bleeding from one of the brain's cerebral arteries can impair blood flow in the brain.

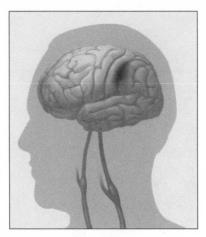

> A part of the brain can be damaged during a stroke.

When blood can't reach the brain for either reason (artery blockage or artery leakage), brain cells begin to die. This is a stroke. Strokes that are caused by blockage are called ischemic strokes. Strokes caused by leakage are hemorrhagic strokes.

Stroke accounted for about 1 of every 15 deaths in the United States in 2003.

Brain damage from a stroke can cause a person to lose certain skills, such as speech or arm or leg movement. Occasionally the brain damage may be so severe that the stroke proves fatal.

If you have been diagnosed with heart disease, you may face an increased risk of stroke. In addition, common types of heart disease such as atrial fibrillation can foster the formation of blood clots—which, if they find their way into arteries of the brain, can trigger strokes.

Recognizing the Symptoms of a Stroke

Because of their vulnerability to stroke, heart-disease patients should learn the symptoms of a stroke—detailed below—and teach them to their friends and family members. Though the effects of a stroke can be severe, prompt medical attention (roughly defined as the first few hours after a stroke) can maximize your degree of recovery.

- Weakness: Be aware of sudden clumsiness or weakness on one side of the body. This is a common stroke symptom.

- Numbness and tingling: A loss of feeling in your face, arm, or leg can signal a stroke. It may feel as if a limb has "fallen asleep."

- Vision problems: A sudden change in vision, double vision, or trouble seeing with one or both eyes could be a stroke symptom.

- Speech or language difficulty: Watch for trouble in talking, slurred speech, or problems understanding others when they speak.

- Imbalance: Stroke symptoms may include dizziness, a sensation of spinning, a loss of balance, and falling down.

- Headache: A sudden, severe headache or migraine may be a sign of stroke.

- Blackouts: Losing consciousness is another stroke symptom. Instruct family members in advance to call 911 immediately should you ever black out.

Heed the Signs of Impending Attack

About 15 percent of stroke victims receive a telltale warning that a stroke may occur in the near future. This alert—called a transient ischemic attack (TIA) or "ministroke"—is brought on by a temporary loss of blood flow to part of the brain. A TIA causes the same symptoms as a stroke but usually lasts for just a few minutes. It typically leaves no lasting damage; people who experience repeated TIAs, however, may suffer permanent brain injury and some loss of mental function from this recurring oxygen deprivation. If you think you are having symptoms of a stroke—even if they don't last—get medical help right away.

About half of all people who experience a TIA fail to report it to their health care provider.

Reducing Your Risk 3

EXCEPT IN RARE INSTANCES, heart disease develops over a period of years with no discernible symptoms—you won't feel like anything is wrong. That means heart disease can be easy to ignore even as it becomes more and more of a threat to your health. But there are ways of determining whether you may be at risk. Decades of scientific research have identified a variety of attributes, conditions, and behaviors that increase your chances of getting heart disease. Some of these so-called risk factors cannot be altered. Others can. The good news is that in either case, no matter what your age, you can take steps to improve your odds.

Aong the risk factors you cannot control are your age, your sex, and your family's medical history of heart disease and related ailments.

Although you can't do anything to change these factors, knowing about the risks they pose should prompt you to increased vigilance, primarily in the form of routine medical checkups and closer monitoring of the factors you can control.

As for the behaviors and habits you can do something about, this chapter provides practical guidance on how to make the kinds of changes in your lifestyle that will lessen your chances of developing atherosclerosis—the buildup of fatty deposits called plaque inside arteries that leads to heart disease and other problems. Even if you've already been diagnosed with heart disease or already had a heart attack, by following the steps outlined here you can significantly improve your chances of avoiding another heart attack, a stroke, or any of the other debilitating effects of America's number one killer.

How Risk Factors Affect the Heart

To function properly, arteries must have smooth, unobstructed linings that allow blood to flow freely so oxygen can reach tissues. Healthy coronary arteries are particularly important because the heart's demand for oxygen varies. During exercise, for example, when the heart is beating harder, more oxygen must reach its tissues and the coronary arteries must be able to meet the rising load.

Some of the risk factors for heart disease—chiefly high blood pressure, stress, and smoking—damage the artery linings and initiate the disease process known as atherosclerosis. Crucial to this process is another major risk factor: elevated levels of the "bad" cholesterol known as LDL, or low-density lipoprotein, in the blood. The result is the buildup of fatty, cholesterol-laden deposits called plaques, which narrow arteries and stiffen them. Diseased arteries restrict blood flow, keeping adequate oxygen from reaching the body's tissues.

Atherosclerosis can strike arteries anywhere in the body and cause problems; a severely restricted artery in the brain, for example, can cause a stroke. In the heart, the effects are especially dangerous. Restricted, inelastic coronary arteries both starve the heart muscle of oxygen and fail to adjust to the heart's varying demands.

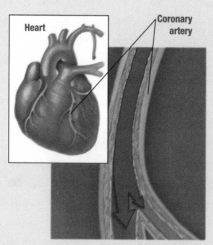

Heart

Coronary artery

> Healthy coronary arteries are elastic and have smooth linings, supplying heart tissue with all the blood it needs. When the lining is damaged and plaque builds up, blood can't flow freely.

Assessing Your Risk

The risk factors for heart disease all contribute to the same thing: the development of atherosclerosis, the underlying process that causes plaque to accumulate in arteries. But not all risk factors are created equal. In addition to being distinguished by whether or not you can control them, risk factors can be more or less virulent, and your own intervention more or less effective in reducing your risk. Some factors are especially pernicious when found in combination.

Risks You Can't Change

- The older you are, the greater your risk. Generally speaking, men over 45 and women over 55 face an elevated risk of developing heart disease, and the risk increases with age after that.
- Being male increases your risk. Although heart disease is the leading cause of death for adults of both sexes, women tend to develop heart disease about 10 years later in life than men do. The female hormone estrogen may help to protect women against heart disease.
- A family history of heart disease and other signs of atherosclerosis such as stroke puts you at a greater risk of developing heart disease.

Risks You Can Control

- Smoking is the most important risk factor you can do something about. Smoking damages the lining of the arteries, inviting plaques to form. Research indicates that smoking makes you up to six times more likely to suffer a heart attack. Smokers are also at higher risk of blood clots and stroke.
- High blood pressure occurs when blood pushes too hard against artery walls, which can damage the lining. High blood pressure raises your risk of developing atherosclerosis but can be controlled with medication or changes in lifestyle.

- Abnormal cholesterol levels make plaque buildup more likely. Your heart disease risk goes up if you don't have enough high-density lipoprotein cholesterol (HDL, or "good" cholesterol), which flushes "bad" low-density lipoprotein cholesterol (LDL) out of arteries. You're also at risk if you have high levels of LDL or triglycerides (another lipid that can accumulate inside arteries).

- Diabetes prevents the body from using sugars and starches properly, which can damage arteries and lead to heart disease. Having diabetes also makes you more likely to suffer a "silent" heart attack—one with no symptoms. Diabetes increases the risk of heart disease in women even more than it does in men.

- Stress and negative emotions such as pent-up anger have been linked to heart disease through a complex biochemical process. Anxiety and depression in the wake of a heart attack or a diagnosis of heart disease can worsen the risk.

- Excess weight makes other heart-disease risk factors, such as diabetes, more likely. Excess weight around the waist or stomach raises that risk the most.

- A lack of physical activity makes you more apt to develop diabetes, high blood pressure, dangerously high cholesterol levels, and excess weight.

Metabolic syndrome means you have three or more heart-disease risk factors such as abdominal obesity, high blood pressure, high cholesterol, and high blood-sugar levels. Having metabolic syndrome puts you at greatly increased risk of heart disease, stroke, and diabetes.

Taking Action against Risk Factors

Once you know your risk factors, you can start working to reduce or even eliminate the ones you can control. This will undoubtedly mean making some changes in your lifestyle—adjustments that may seem overwhelming at first, especially when they involve altering habits or behaviors that have become second nature. The key is to make changes gradually, starting with one or two at first. When you've mastered those, try making others.

In some cases, medical intervention may be needed to help you control risk factors. You may need medication—to bring down your blood pressure, for example, to lower your blood-cholesterol level, or to keep diabetes in check. But even if your doctor is treating you, there are things you can do yourself to address these problems.

The following pages discuss the main heart-disease risk factors more fully, explaining why they are dangerous and what you can do to manage them.

Damn the Torpor!

If you are physically inactive, you're threatening your heart in more ways than one. Physical inactivity tends to lead to overeating, and the two combined can cause obesity, high levels of LDL cholesterol, and diabetes—all of which raise your heart-disease risk.

Once you've developed heart disease, your heart is essentially out of shape, and intense or unaccustomed exertion—such as running to catch a bus or shoveling snow—can bring on a heart attack or other dangerous consequences as the heart muscle calls for more oxygen than the coronary arteries can supply. You need to increase your level of physical activity cautiously and under your doctor's supervision if you've already got heart disease.

Of Rigor and Routine

Becoming more active will improve your heart's health in many ways. Physical activity can help you lose weight, lower your blood pressure, manage cholesterol levels, and reduce stress. Regular exercise carries the added bonus of strengthening bones and muscles, improving your sleep patterns, and helping you think more clearly.

Try to do 30 minutes of physical activity at least three days a week (or, better yet, every day). Adding just a bit of exercise to your daily routine here and there can help. You don't need fancy equipment to get started. In fact, walking is one of the best ways to work out.

Ideas for Getting Started

Perhaps the best motivator for becoming more physically active is to keep the many benefits of exercise in mind. First and foremost, you'll be improving your cardiovascular health. But you'll also look and feel better, and you will have more energy.

It's important to recognize that you're more likely to stick with something you like. Talk with your health care provider about the physical activities you want to try. Start with the ones you think you'll enjoy most. You could try:

- Walking, by yourself or with friends. You can walk indoors if you prefer. Some shopping malls and schools open early to accommodate walkers.
- Joining an exercise class or gym. Not all gyms are expensive. Many people find working out with others more enjoyable and more motivating than exercising alone.
- Using exercise or aerobics videos.
- Swimming laps at a local pool.
- Joining a cardiac rehab program (if you have already been diagnosed with heart disease). Ask your health care provider to help you find a suitable program. You can also call the American Association of Cardiovascular and Pulmonary Rehabilitation at 312-321-5146 or visit that organization online at www.aacvpr.org.

Yes, You Can Find the Time

You may be surprised at how easy it is to incorporate some additional form of physical activity into your day. For example, you can:

- Climb the stairs instead of riding the elevator.
- Park your car a little farther from the store.
- Join your children or grandchildren's game of tag.
- Walk your dog a little farther than usual.
- Seize any and every opportunity to walk—to a friend's house, say, or to the store—instead of driving.
- Use a bathroom on another floor at work or at home (and take the stairs to get there).

- Walk the entire grocery store boustrophedonically—a fancy word for "up one aisle and down the next."
- Tackle an extra household chore, such as scrubbing the floor or vacuuming.
- Work in the garden.

It's perfectly all right to get your daily exercise in several brief stints rather than one sustained effort. Short periods of exercise quickly add up: Five minutes of stair climbing, 10 minutes of vacuuming, and 15 minutes of gardening, for example, satisfy your 30 daily exercise minutes.

High Blood Pressure

High blood pressure, also called hypertension, is known as the "silent killer" because it often has no symptoms. The only way to find out whether you have it is to get your blood pressure checked. Left uncontrolled, high blood pressure can lead to heart disease, heart attack, stroke, kidney disease, or blindness.

Blood pressure is a measurement of the force with which blood presses against the inside walls of the arteries. It is recorded as millimeters of mercury (mm Hg) because blood pressure was once measured with a glass device filled with mercury and marked off in millimeters.

Your blood pressure is too high if it consistently measures more than 120/80 mm Hg ("120 over 80"). The top number, the systolic pressure, denotes the pressure created in your arteries when your heart pumps. The bottom number, the diastolic pressure, reflects the arterial pressure between heartbeats. See the chart on page 40 for specific ranges. The standards for people with diabetes are different, with values at or above 130 systolic considered hypertensive.

The more risk factors you have, the greater your chances of developing heart disease. Eliminating whatever risks you can is therefore vitally important.

Rarely do blood-pressure problems go away on their own. But making some lifestyle changes and taking prescribed medication can help lower elevated readings to normal levels.

Compare your blood pressure to the ranges in this chart. Is your blood pressure at a healthy level?			
Number	**Normal**	**Prehypertensive**	**Hypertension**
Top (systolic)	Below 120	120-139	140 or higher
Bottom (diastolic)	Below 80	80-89	90 or higher

Pounding Exacts Its Toll

When blood pressure is too high, the abnormally intense pounding of blood in arteries gradually damages them. It wears away the smooth inner lining, providing a roughened surface where plaque can form. Affected arteries thicken, lose their elasticity, and become less efficient at transporting blood. The diminished blood flow then damages the organs nourished by the arteries—the heart, brain, kidneys, eyes, and others.

High-Pressure Perils

When high blood pressure damages artery walls, the risk of the following health problems increases.

- Coronary artery disease: If the arteries that bring blood to the heart muscle are damaged, heart tissue may not get enough oxygen. This can lead to angina and other heart problems.
- Heart attack: If a coronary artery becomes blocked—either by the buildup of plaque or by the formation of a blood clot—it cuts off blood flow, killing that part of the heart muscle it should supply. The result is a heart attack.

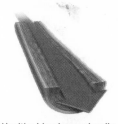

Healthy blood-vessel walls allow blood to flow freely.

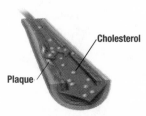

Damaged blood-vessel walls make it easier for cholesterol to adhere and form plaques.

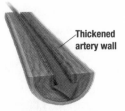

The blood-vessel walls thicken. This narrows the vessel and curbs blood flow.

- Stroke: Severely constricted or blocked blood flow to part of the brain causes a stroke by preventing oxygen from reaching those brain cells.
- Heart failure: When arteries narrow, the heart has to work harder to force blood through them. This can cause the heart muscle to thicken or the heart to enlarge; the heart may then fail to work as well as it should.
- Other problems: High blood pressure can damage the myriad small arteries supplying blood to the kidneys and the retinas, leading to kidney disease or blindness. If damaged arteries reduce blood flow to the legs, you may experience leg pain and swelling during physical activity.

Taking Your Blood Pressure

You can track your blood pressure easily and painlessly. Many people use the do-it-yourself monitors available at some grocery stores and pharmacies. If you're being treated for high blood pressure, your health care provider will probably ask you to measure your blood pressure at home. Here's how to do it using an at-home digital monitor.

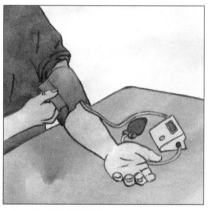

> Position the blood-pressure cuff, and keep it level with your heart.

1. **Relax**
   - If you just ate, exercised, or smoked, wait at least 30 minutes before taking a reading.
   - Sit comfortably with your arm on a table, palm up. Place the monitor near you.
   - Rest a few minutes before you begin.

2. **Wrap the Cuff**
   - Wrap the cuff around your upper arm, just above your elbow. This is best done on bare skin, not over clothing.
   - Make sure the cuff is at the level of your heart.

3. **Inflate the Cuff**
   - If you have a self-inflating cuff, push the button that starts the pump. Otherwise, pump up the cuff until the monitor reads the pressure recommended by your health care provider, then stop pumping.
   - The cuff will then slowly loosen, and the numbers on the monitor will rapidly change. When they stop changing, your blood-pressure reading will appear.

4. **Record the Results**
   - Write down your blood-pressure numbers. Note the date and time. Some newer at-home monitors store readings automatically, allowing you to look them up later.
   - Remove the cuff from your arm. Turn off the machine.

Tips for Accurate Results

- Ask your health care provider to help you decide which type of monitor is best for you.
- Read and follow the instructions for your monitor carefully, especially with a model that is new to you.
- If you get a reading that is uncharacteristically high or low, relax for a few minutes. Then repeat the test.
- Take readings as often as your health care provider recommends. Be consistent about the timing and circumstances.

To Lower Your Blood Pressure

People with prehypertension or mild hypertension—when the heart valves are at or just above the threshold defining hypertension—can often lower their pressure into the normal range without medication. Here are some good ways to start.

Exercise regularly

Couch potatoes are much more susceptible to hypertension and its consequences than people who are physically active. If you already have high blood pressure, engaging in regular exercise can help lower it. Slowly work up to at least 30 minutes of physical activity a day. Talk to your doctor before beginning any exercise program.

Lose weight

Carrying extra pounds forces your heart to work harder. Losing weight—and keeping it off—is one of the most important things you can do to lower your blood pressure. Shedding just a few pounds can reduce blood pressure significantly.

Stop smoking

Smoking is the leading cause of illness and death in the United States and one of the major risk factors for heart disease. In addition to raising blood pressure, it encourages the formation of blood clots that can trigger heart attacks, and it damages blood vessels. The benefits of quitting are strikingly clear: Just three years after kicking the habit, former smokers have a heart-attack risk close to that of people who have never smoked.

Eat healthier

Limit the amount of fat and salt in your diet. Doing so helps reduce blood pressure—and, by controlling cholesterol levels, helps prevent plaque buildup. Federal guidelines recommend limiting sodium intake to 2.4 grams per day (the amount contained in about one teaspoon of table salt). Americans on average take in between 3.3 and 6 grams of sodium per day, which partly explains the prevalence of hypertension in the United States. Also, try to eat more fruits and vegetables: Studies indicate that a diet rich in produce helps reduce blood pressure in people with hypertension.

Limit alcohol

Although research indicates that moderate amounts of alcohol can be good for your cardiovascular health, too much alcohol can increase blood pressure. Men should limit themselves to no more than 1 ounce of alcohol a day (about two drinks). Women absorb alcohol more readily than men, so they should have no more than half an ounce (one drink).

Reduce stress

Chronic stress can raise blood pressure. To ease stress, get enough sleep, exercise regularly, practice relaxation techniques, and spend more time with your family and friends.

Medication

Lifestyle changes alone may not suffice to keep your blood pressure at a safe level. Fortunately, blood-pressure medications developed over the past 20 years are able to control virtually all cases of hypertension. In order for any blood pressure medication to work, however, you must be sure to use it properly:

- Take the medicine each day or as your doctor directs.
- Do not skip doses or stop taking your medication without your doctor's okay.
- Talk to your doctor about what to do if you miss a dose.

High Blood Cholesterol

Cholesterol is a naturally occurring fatty substance manufactured by the body to build new cells, insulate nerves, and produce hormones. It is also present in some foods, primarily meats, dairy products, and shellfish. High levels of cholesterol in the bloodstream can lead to heart disease and other vascular problems, especially for people who have other risk factors associated with the development of athero-

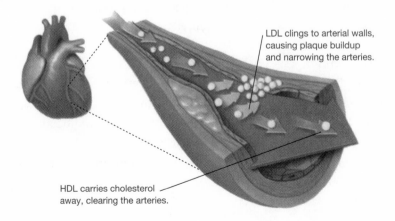

LDL clings to arterial walls, causing plaque buildup and narrowing the arteries.

HDL carries cholesterol away, clearing the arteries.

Your health care practitioner can check your cholesterol with a simple blood test after you have been fasting (nothing to eat or drink) for 12 hours. The results include numbers for total cholesterol, LDL, HDL, and the blood fats called triglycerides, which can also lead to blocked arteries.

- Total cholesterol: This number includes LDL and HDL cholesterol, plus other fats in the bloodstream. Your total should be less than 200. A total from 200 to 239 is borderline high, and readings of 240 or more indicate you have high cholesterol.

  My total cholesterol is: _____

- LDL: A number below 130 is good; between 130 and 160 is borderline; and 160 or above is high. For people with heart disease or diabetes, LDL cholesterol should be 70 or less.

  My LDL cholesterol is: _____

- HDL: HDL cholesterol should be 40 or higher for men, 50 or higher for women.

  My HDL cholesterol is: _____

- Triglycerides: Triglycerides are fatty substances in the blood that, like cholesterol, can lead to blocked arteries. Your triglyceride level should be less than 150.

  My triglyceride level is: _____

- Ratio: Your results may also include a number indicating the ratio of total cholesterol to HDL. Any number below 4 is good. For men, anywhere from 4.2 to 7.3 is acceptable; for women, from 3.9 to 5.7.

  My ratio is: _____

sclerosis. Knowing your cholesterol levels—and understanding the distinction between "good" HDL cholesterol and "bad" LDL cholesterol—is a vital first step toward making any necessary changes to reduce your risk.

Cholesterol: The Good, the Bad, and the Fatty

The human body produces all the cholesterol it needs in the liver, which releases it into the bloodstream. Protein molecules then bind with cholesterol to form two different kinds of particles known as lipoproteins. Low-density lipoproteins (LDL) are relatively large molecules that tend to remain in the bloodstream; this is the so-called "bad" form of cholesterol. High-density lipoproteins (HDL) are compact particles that remove excess cholesterol from the bloodstream, carrying it to the liver where it is broken down and then expelled; this is the "good" cholesterol.

High levels of LDL or low levels of HDL—or, as often occurs, a combination of both—lead to the development of atherosclerosis as excess cholesterol carried by LDL particles infiltrates arterial walls and begins forming plaque deposits.

Strategies to Control Cholesterol

A diet high in saturated fats encourages the liver to produce more cholesterol than the body needs; dietary cholesterol also contributes to the problem. And trans-fatty acids—artificially produced fats found in many processed foods—have the particularly nasty effect of both raising levels of "bad" LDL cholesterol and lowering levels of "good" HDL cholesterol.

Reducing your blood-cholesterol level by 25 percent cuts your risk of heart attack in half.

If your cholesterol levels are out of whack, you can take steps to bring them to appropriate levels. If your levels are normal, you should learn how to keep them that way. Eating the right foods and getting enough exercise are the most important things you can do. Some people also require medication to control their cholesterol levels.

Moving toward Better Cholesterol Levels

Read through the following checklist. It can help you learn whether or not you're controlling your cholesterol and what you can do to improve your numbers. Put a check mark before each statement that is true for you.

☐ Whole grains, pasta, and cereals are a large part of my diet.
☐ I choose low-fat or nonfat dairy products and lean cuts of meat.

• **Eat Less Saturated Fat.** This type of fat does the most harm because the body turns it into cholesterol. Saturated fats are found mainly in animal products such as meat, poultry skin, cheese, whole milk, and butter. Coconut oil, cocoa butter, palm-kernel oil, and palm oil are also saturated fats. To reduce your saturated-fat intake, choose lean meats, skinless poultry, and fish that is baked or broiled rather than fried. And limit your intake of each of these foods to no more than 6 ounces per day.

• **Eat Less Dietary Cholesterol.** Cholesterol in your diet increases the level of cholesterol in your bloodstream. Dietary cholesterol is found only in foods that come from animals. Sources include eggs and other dairy products, liver, meats, and shellfish.

• **Eat More Fiber.** Eating enough fiber can help reduce blood cholesterol. Important sources include oats, dried beans, brown rice, vegetables, and fruit.

• **Be Physically Active.** Staying physically active raises your good cholesterol (HDL). It also helps you lose weight, which can lower your bad cholesterol (LDL). Walking, swimming, and cycling are all excellent forms of exercise. Check with your doctor before starting any program of physical activity. You might begin with three 10-minute sessions on most days of the week, then slowly work up to at least 30 minutes at a time every day.

• **Take Your Medication.** If diet and exercise do not lower your cholesterol enough, your doctor may prescribe medication. Be sure to take it as directed.

☐ I eat at least five servings of fruits and vegetables daily.
☐ I rarely eat fast foods, deep-fried foods, or packaged baked goods.
☐ I exercise at least 30 minutes most days.
☐ My body weight is about right (see chart, page 53).
☐ My cholesterol was checked within the last couple of years and was normal.

The more check marks you made, the better you are doing at controlling your cholesterol. If you need to improve your numbers, use any statements you didn't check as a goal to work on. Then take the quiz again in two months to see how much progress you've made.

Cigarette Smoking

Smoking should be Public Enemy No. 1: It is the leading cause of preventable deaths among Americans, killing more than 400,000 people a year. Although 140,000 of these deaths stem from lung cancer, at least one-third are related to heart disease.

Smoking contributes to heart disease in a number of ways:

- Nicotine, carbon monoxide, and other compounds in cigarette smoke (there are nearly 4,000 of them) trigger atherosclerosis by damaging artery linings. Cholesterol is then attracted to the injured areas and plaque builds up.
- Smoking reduces the proportion of good (HDL) cholesterol to bad (LDL) cholesterol in the blood.
- The nicotine in cigarette smoke raises blood pressure.
- Cigarette smoke causes blood to clot more readily, potentially obstructing blood flow. Clots can cause heart attacks and strokes.
- Carbon monoxide in cigarette smoke latches onto red blood cells, reducing the amount of oxygen they can carry to the heart and the rest of the body.
- Smoking can cause arteries to contract or spasm, curtailing blood flow.

Gauging Your Risk from Smoking

The more cigarettes you smoke a day and the longer you have smoked, the greater your risk of coronary artery disease. Smoking just four cigarettes a day increases your risk of heart attack by 50 percent over that of a nonsmoker. One pack a day doubles your risk. And if you smoke two or more packs a day, your disease risk becomes three times higher than it is for a person who has never smoked.

Here's How to Lower Your Risk

If you're a smoker, the best way to lower your risk of heart disease is simple to understand but can be devilishly difficult to accomplish: Quit. You can cut down gradually or you can quit "cold turkey." Motivate yourself by listing your reasons for quitting. Focus on the positive: Think what it will be like to taste food again, or to walk up stairs without gasping for breath. You can also calculate how much money you will save!

> A smoker's risk of heart attack is more than twice that of a nonsmoker.

Seeking assistance through a smoking-cessation clinic or a support group may help you kick the habit. You can also ask your doctor about stop-smoking aids. The reward will be as precious as life itself: Three short years after you quit, your risk of heart attack will have dropped to near normal.

Metabolic Syndrome

An estimated 47 million Americans have a cluster of several heart-disease risk factors that dramatically increases their risk for heart disease, stroke, and diabetes. According to the most widely accepted definition, someone has metabolic syndrome if they develop three or more of the following conditions:

- Abdominal obesity. This is defined as a waist size of 40 or more inches for men and more than 35 inches for women.
- Elevated blood sugar. This is usually a sign of insulin resistance, where sugar levels in the blood rise because cells become less sensitive to insulin (the hormone that moves sugar into cells so it can be used for energy). Insulin resistance is called a "prediabetic" condition because many people who have it go on to develop type 2 diabetes.
- High triglyceride levels. Triglyceride is the fat most commonly found in the blood and at high levels can contribute to the development of atherosclerosis.
- Low levels of HDL ("good") cholesterol. (See recommended levels of HDL for men and women on page 45.)

- High levels of LDL ("bad") cholesterol.
- High blood pressure. (See discussion of high blood pressure on pages 39–46.)

People who have metabolic syndrome should be under a doctor's care so that the syndrome's various risk factors can be closely monitored. Controlling these risk factors may require medication. But there are also things that *you* can do to treat the condition. In particular, exercising and adopting a low-fat, healthy diet can help you lose weight. These two simple steps attack metabolic syndrome on several other fronts, since they help decrease insulin resistance, lower blood pressure and triglyceride levels, and raise HDL levels. Chapter 5 describes strategies for adopting a healthy diet and an enjoyable exercise regimen.

Diabetes

Diabetes, a major health problem in itself, can also be a "hidden" heart-disease risk: Many people with this disease don't initially know they have it. If you have diabetes, your coronary arteries may become damaged more easily, leading to atherosclerosis. You are

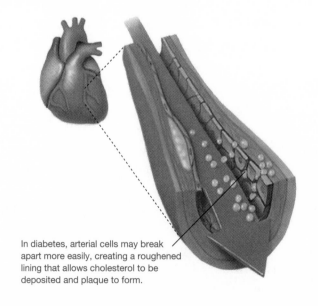

In diabetes, arterial cells may break apart more easily, creating a roughened lining that allows cholesterol to be deposited and plaque to form.

more likely to have other risk factors, such as high blood cholesterol, high blood pressure, and obesity.

Type 2 diabetes is the most common form. It usually appears in adults, often in middle age, but is more and more prevalent in adolescents—and even in children. People who are overweight and physically inactive are the most likely to develop type 2 diabetes.

Damage from Diabetes

Diabetes prevents the body from using sugars and starches properly. As a result, arteries may be damaged more easily because the "cement" binding cells in the blood-vessel walls is weaker. This damage increases the risk for atherosclerosis and heart disease.

Measuring Your Diabetes Risk

Simple blood tests (blood glucose or sugar tolerance tests) can tell you if you have diabetes or are likely to get it. A medical evaluation can also help uncover diabetes. Are you overweight or constantly thirsty? Do you urinate frequently? These are among the most common symptoms of diabetes.

If you have diabetes, you can help control its effects by keeping your blood-sugar levels normal. Work with your health care team to design an eating plan to regulate your blood sugar. If changing the way you eat fails to control your diabetes, your doctor may prescribe medications or insulin—a commercially prepared hormone designed to manage blood-sugar levels. To lower other risks, lose extra pounds with exercise and by limiting foods high in fat or cholesterol.

Being Overweight

People who carry excess body fat—especially at the waist—have an increased risk of developing heart disease even if they have no other risk factors.

Excess weight contributes to heart disease in several ways. It raises blood pressure, total blood cholesterol, and triglyceride levels;

lowers levels of good (HDL) cholesterol; and makes people more likely to develop type 2 diabetes.

Those extra pounds also force the heart to work harder, boosting its need for oxygen. This can make a heart attack more likely, especially if atherosclerosis has already narrowed coronary arteries with plaque and reduced blood flow to the heart muscle.

Of all the risk factors for heart disease, being overweight may be the simplest to do something about. By combining a healthy diet with regular exercise, you can lose weight and keep it off. Even modest weight loss can be helpful: You can lower your heart-disease risk by shedding as few as 10 pounds.

Are You Overweight?

There's a standard way to tell if you're overweight: Calculate your body mass index (BMI), a number that gauges your weight as a function of your height. To find your BMI, consult the BMI chart on page 53. First find your height and weight, then circle the number where they meet; this is your BMI. If you're 5'4" and weigh 180 pounds, for example, your BMI is 31. If you lost 10 pounds, your BMI would fall to 29. (You can also calculate your BMI as follows: Divide your weight in pounds by the square of your height in inches, then multiply the result by 703.)

About two-thirds of American adults can be classified as overweight. More than a quarter are considered obese.

It's best to keep your BMI between 19 and 25. If your BMI is 25 or above, you should lose some weight. A BMI of 25 to 29.9 puts you in the "overweight" category; people with a BMI of 30 or above are considered obese.

Make a Plan to Lose Weight

The safest and most effective way to lose weight involves two steps: Consuming fewer calories and becoming more physically active. Though you may lose weight quickly with a "fad" diet or one that severely restricts your calories, you'll likely put the weight right back on—and you may risk your health in the process.

Talk to your health care provider or a dietitian to set some realistic weight-loss goals, then discuss safe ways to achieve them. One

Weight

(lb)	120	130	140	150	160	170	180	190	200	210	220	230	240	250	260	270	280	290	300	310	320
5'0"	23	25	27	29	31	33	35	37	39	41	42	44	47	49	51	53	55	57	59	61	62
5'1"	23	25	26	28	31	33	35	37	39	41	42	44	47	49	51	53	55	57	59	61	62
5'2"	22	24	26	27	29	31	33	35	37	38	40	42	44	46	48	49	51	53	55	57	59
5'3"	21	23	25	27	28	30	32	34	35	37	39	41	43	44	46	48	50	51	53	55	57
5'4"	21	22	24	26	27	29	31	33	34	36	38	39	41	43	45	46	48	50	51	53	55
5'5"	20	22	23	25	27	28	30	32	33	35	37	38	40	42	43	45	47	48	50	52	53
5'6"	19	21	23	24	26	27	29	31	32	34	36	37	39	40	42	44	45	47	48	50	52
5'7"	19	20	22	23	25	27	28	30	31	33	34	36	38	39	40	42	44	45	47	49	50
5'8"	18	20	21	23	24	26	27	29	30	32	33	35	36	38	40	41	43	44	46	47	49
5'9"	18	19	21	22	24	25	27	28	30	31	32	34	35	37	38	40	41	43	44	46	47
5'10"	17	19	20	22	23	24	26	27	29	30	32	33	34	36	37	39	40	42	43	44	46
5'11"	17	18	20	21	22	24	25	26	28	29	31	32	33	35	36	38	39	40	42	43	45
6'0"	16	18	19	20	22	23	24	26	27	28	30	31	33	34	35	37	38	39	41	42	43
6'1"	16	18	19	20	21	22	24	25	26	28	29	30	32	33	34	36	37	38	40	41	42
6'2"	15	17	18	19	21	22	23	24	26	27	28	30	31	32	33	35	36	37	39	40	41
6'3"	15	16	18	19	20	21	23	24	25	26	28	29	30	31	33	34	35	36	38	39	40
6'4"	15	16	17	18	19	21	22	23	24	26	27	28	29	30	32	33	34	35	37	38	39

Height

My BMI: ____________

Key: Normal weight (BMI 19 to 25) Overweight (BMI 26 to 29) Obese (BMI 30 or over)

common weight-loss goal is to lose 1 pound a week until you reach your target. Simple adjustments may help you achieve your goal: switching from whole milk to skim, for instance, or from regular soda to diet. In tandem with your dietary changes, follow the tips on pages 37–39 to add physical activity to your daily routine.

The Dangers of Stress

Being under stress makes your blood pressure soar and your heart rate rise, both of which can damage the lining of your arteries.

All of us routinely confront stressful situations in our lives. How we react to those circumstances determines the degree of risk we face. Research has shown that heart attacks are more common in people who react to stressful situations in an angry, hostile way. The key is to know what triggers your stress response (see sidebar, page 54), then find ways to avoid those triggers or deal with them in a calm, relaxed manner. Eating well, exercising, and getting enough sleep are also proven stress busters.

Take some time to think about your stress triggers and how you react to them. You might try keeping a stress diary for a few week, which not only will help you enumerate your triggers but may also reveal that you fall into unhealthy habits when you're under stress—such as eating poorly, smoking, or skipping exercise.

Don't bank on being able to eliminate all your stress triggers, but you'll almost certainly be able to do *something* about most of them. For example, contending with rush-hour traffic causes many people to react negatively, and it can be hard to avoid the situation. But you can minimize its emotional impact on you. Instead of getting steamed up during the morning rush, use the time in your car to listen to an audiobook or to classical music on the radio. Or see if leaving home 10 minutes earlier allows you to avoid some traffic. Even small changes like these can make a difference and help you feel more in control of your life.

Target Your Triggers

Many everyday situations—especially those listed below—can trigger a stress response. See which of your own stress triggers you can defuse.

Getting stuck in traffic
Waiting in line
Running late
Forgetting or losing things
Coming home to a messy house
Arguing with family, friends, or coworkers
Juggling demands on your time
Having money or credit problems

Stress and Your Heart

Did you know?

- Stress causes the body to release hormones that make the heart pump harder and faster.
- Chronic stress makes the blood vessels narrower. This can cause blood pressure to rise.
- Stress can damage the lining of the arteries, which in turn causes plaque to form. This reduces blood flow and may damage the heart.

Managing stress helps reduce your health risks.

- It may help lower blood pressure and cholesterol.
- It can help you stop smoking.
- Other benefits: It can help you sleep better, have more energy, and be better able to handle the ups and downs of daily life.

Summarizing Your Risk Factors

After reading this chapter, you should have a fairly solid idea of whether you are at risk of developing heart disease. Now it's time to add up those risks so that you can assess the severity of the risk you face.

Listed on pages 56 and 57 are the most important risk factors for heart disease. Check "yes" for those that apply to you or "no" for those that don't. Go through the list again in a few months to see if you've reduced your risks.

Your Risk Factors

High-Fat Diet   Yes   No

Do you eat fatty meats or "fast foods" on most days?   ___ ___

Do you often eat high-fat dairy products such as   ___ ___
butter, cheese, and ice cream?

Do you eat more processed, packaged foods   ___ ___
than grains, fruits, and vegetables?

High Blood Cholesterol

Is you total blood cholesterol 200 or higher?   ___ ___

Is your LDL ("bad") cholesterol 100 or higher?   ___ ___

Lack of Exercise

Do you exercise fewer than 3 times a week?   ___ ___

Do you sit down to do your work?   ___ ___

Is most of your recreation done sitting down?   ___ ___

Excess Weight

Is your body-mass index (BMI) in an unhealthy range?   ___ ___

(See page 53 to calculate your BMI.)   ___ ___

Smoking

Do you smoke or chew tobacco?   ___ ___

Have you tried to quit?   ___ ___

Diabetes

Do you or other family members have diabetes?   ___ ___

If you have diabetes, is your blood sugar often high?   ___ ___

High Blood Pressure

Is your blood pressure higher than 120/80?   ___ ___

Do you often choose salty foods?   ___ ___

Stress

	Yes	No
Do you avoid talking to others when you're upset?	__	__
Do you often feel nervous or depressed?	__	__
Do you often feel angry about things that are beyond your control?	__	__

Family History

	Yes	No
Do you have a male relative who had heart disease when he was 55 or younger?	__	__
Do you have a female relative who had heart disease when she was 65 or younger?	__	__

Other Risk Factors

	Yes	No
Are you a man older than 45, or a woman over 55?	__	__
Has your doctor said you have other risk factors for heart disease?	__	__

Your Results

The more times you answered "Yes," the higher your risk for a heart attack or stroke. You can begin to lower your chances of developing heart disease and other problems by eliminating or otherwise controlling as many of these risk factors as you can. Assess your progress every few months.

	Date	Number of "yes" answers
Today:	_____	_____
3 months later	_____	_____
6 months later	_____	_____

Do You Have Heart Disease? 4

T HE NUMBERS ARE STAGGERING: Half a million Americans a year die of heart attacks, and nearly a million more undergo serious surgical procedures to treat advanced cases of heart disease. Just as stunning, though, is how often these devastating circumstances could be averted.

It's best, of course, to prevent heart disease from occurring in the first place by knowing the risk factors and making appropriate changes to your lifestyle. But it's equally important to be able to recognize the symptoms of heart disease when it has already developed. Early detection—and prompt action—is the key to preventing this killer disease from doing its worst.

This chapter describes the most common symptoms that provide an early warning of heart disease. It also details the medical exams and diagnostic tests that can confirm the presence of heart disease and assess its severity.

When Symptoms Matter

In simplest terms, a symptom is a change in the way your body feels that indicates the presence of a disease or other health problem. It's not always easy to gauge whether a symptom should lead you to seek medical attention. Indeed, some of the symptoms of heart disease are similar to the sorts of everyday aches and pains that signal no serious underlying problem. Generally, however, you should think about contacting your health care professional if a symptom you suspect might be related to heart disease has any of the following characteristics:

- You have never had the symptom before.
- The pain is severe.
- The symptom is getting worse and makes you feel anxious.
- Medications you've been taking fail to relieve the problem.
- The symptom forces you to curtail a physical activity—slowing you to a walk if you've been running, for example.
- You've already had a heart attack and had this symptom before.

Chest Pain: Is It Heart Disease?

Chest pain is the symptom most commonly associated with heart disease, but it doesn't always indicate a problem with the heart itself. Sometimes the cause may be a serious condition affecting the aorta or even the stomach. Often, though, pain in the chest stems from more mundane problems, such as a pulled muscle in the chest wall, strained rib cartilage, or heartburn caused by stomach acid that backs up, or refluxes, into the esophagus.

One particular type of chest pain should never be ignored: A steady, squeezing, or crushing pain in the middle of the chest that lasts longer than two minutes could signal a heart attack. Many people who have suffered fatal heart attacks might have been saved had they not incorrectly assumed that the pain was caused by something else and delayed seeking treatment.

Because chest pain has a number of different causes, it's best to let your health care provider determine whether it's related to heart disease.

The Telltale Pain of Angina

More than 200 years ago, British physician William Heberden coined the term "angina pectoris"—literally, a strangling of the chest—to describe what is now considered the classic symptom of coronary artery disease. Doctors today typically refer to it simply as angina, in part because the pain doesn't always occur in the chest.

Like every other muscle in the body, the heart needs an adequate supply of oxygen to function properly. But when heart disease narrows the coronary arteries, too little blood—and therefore too

When Chest Pain Means Heart Attack

A heart attack occurs when plaque or a blood clot blocks a coronary artery for a significant amount of time—permanently or anywhere from 30 minutes to two hours. When oxygen-rich blood can't reach heart-muscle tissue, that part of the heart muscle dies—and the damage is irreversible. Myocardial infarction, the technical term for heart attack, literally means a region of cell death within the myocardium (heart muscle).

Heart-attack symptoms are similar to those for angina, but they are typically more severe and last longer than two minutes. The classic symptoms of a heart attack include:

- A feeling of uncomfortable pressure, fullness, squeezing, aching, or pain, usually in the middle of the chest
- Pain, aching, or heaviness in the shoulders, neck, jaw, arms, or upper back (or that spreads to those areas from the chest)
- Pain accompanied by lightheadedness, sweating, nausea, vomiting, shortness of breath, or fainting

If you experience any of these symptoms, call an ambulance immediately or ask someone to rush you to the nearest hospital. If possible, take a standard (325 mg) aspirin tablet right away. Aspirin has blood-thinning properties and can help stop any clots from growing larger.

Many people survive heart attacks, especially when they receive prompt medical attention. Tragically, though, half of all heart-attack victims wait more than two hours before going to a hospital—usually because they don't know they're having a heart attack. Studies suggest that treatment with potent clot-dissolving drugs within two hours of the first symptoms could prevent as many as 90 percent of heart-attack deaths. Emergency angioplasty—in which a balloon at the tip of a catheter is inflated to widen a blocked artery (see Chapter 6)—might be even more effective.

little oxygen—reaches the heart muscle. This is especially so during physical exertion or moments of great anxiety, when the heart beats harder and faster. The lack of an adequate blood supply stimulates nerves in the heart muscle, causing pain.

It's important to understand that anginal pain is not a heart attack, nor does it cause lasting damage to the heart. But it does indicate the presence of coronary artery disease, by far the most common type of heart ailment. And it also means you are at risk of having a heart attack. In fact, angina makes you four to five times more likely to suffer a heart attack. So if you've been diagnosed with angina, think of it as a wake-up call to take aggressive and immediate action.

For one thing, you need to modify your risk factors for heart disease, as discussed in Chapter 3. You can also take steps to relieve your symptoms and live an active life; Chapter 6 describes treatment options for angina.

Angina symptoms vary from person to person, but they generally remain consistent from one episode to the next.

Here's how angina might feel:

- You may experience pain, heaviness, tightness, pressure, burning, or aching in the middle of your chest.
- These symptoms also occur in the chest, back, neck, throat, or jaw, or in the arms, elbows, wrists, or shoulders.
- You may also have other symptoms at the same time, such as tiredness, nausea, sweating, shortness of breath, lightheadedness, increased heart rate, or an irregular heart rate.
- Women with angina frequently feel neck, shoulder, or mid-back pain; nausea; indigestion; fatigue; dizziness; palpitations; or shortness of breath.

Doctors distinguish between two kinds of angina:

- Stable angina occurs at predictable times, usually when you're doing something active such as climbing stairs; anger or stress may trigger it as well. Resting—or calming down and relaxing—relieves the symptoms of stable angina within a few minutes.
- Unstable angina is not predictable and can occur at any time, even during rest; attacks also tend to last longer. Unstable angina is more serious than stable angina and is a sign that a heart attack is likely in the near future. Variant angina—a type of unstable angina—happens when a coronary artery goes into spasm. Two-thirds of people with variant angina have severely restricted blood flow in at least one coronary artery.

Angina and the Progression of Heart Disease

The pain of angina is a response to heart disease that is developing, and the type of angina—stable or unstable—reflects the degree to which the disease has progressed.

The process begins when one or more of the risk factors for heart disease—such as smoking, stress, or high blood pressure—damages the inner lining of coronary arteries. This sets the stage for atherosclerosis: the buildup of plaque deposits and the formation of scar tissue, which not only narrows the channel through which blood flows but also stiffens the arteries' walls and makes them less able to expand.

An early sign of trouble is so-called stable angina, which occurs when the heart needs extra oxygen but narrowed, stiffened coronary arteries can't supply it. It's known as stable angina because it tends to happen at predictable times, such as during physical exertion. As heart disease progresses, plaque builds up even more and sometimes ruptures, forming blood clots. When a clot or accumulated plaque severely restricts blood flow, the resulting anginal pain is called unstable because it occurs unpredictably, even at rest. If an artery becomes completely blocked, the result is a heart attack.

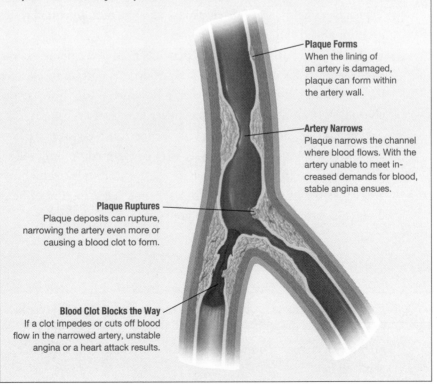

Plaque Forms
When the lining of an artery is damaged, plaque can form within the artery wall.

Artery Narrows
Plaque narrows the channel where blood flows. With the artery unable to meet increased demands for blood, stable angina ensues.

Plaque Ruptures
Plaque deposits can rupture, narrowing the artery even more or causing a blood clot to form.

Blood Clot Blocks the Way
If a clot impedes or cuts off blood flow in the narrowed artery, unstable angina or a heart attack results.

Both types of angina need to be treated. If you have had angina for less than six months and aren't sure what brings on an episode, your doctor may treat it as unstable until it is shown to be stable. Call your doctor right away if your angina starts to occur more often or less predictably, lasts longer, or causes more discomfort.

Syncope (aka Fainting)

Maybe you woke up on the ground, embarrassed and scared—perhaps even injured. Or you stood up too quickly, felt lightheaded, and passed out for a moment or two. Why did you faint? Is this a sign of a serious health problem? Fainting, known in medical terminology as syncope, has many different causes, some of which are of major concern. But syncope can also denote an underlying heart condition that you need to address.

Though syncope happens suddenly, certain warning signs may telegraph that it is coming on. These include dimmed vision, lightheadedness, or a rapid heartbeat. But you may get no warning at all. Typically, you'll regain consciousness quickly, though you may feel tired for a while afterward.

Syncope is fairly common. It may mean no more than that you were standing for too long; that you sat up or stood up too fast; or that your blood-sugar level was temporarily too low (hypoglycemia). In some cases, you may never faint again.

But you should also report a loss of consciousness to your physician, who will investigate precisely why you fainted. Among the serious causes is an irregular heart rhythm (arrhythmia), which can also cause the heart to stop. If your syncope is a symptom of heart disease, treatment may even save your life.

Understanding Syncope

Every part of your body needs a steady supply of oxygen-rich blood—including, of course, your brain. To satisfy that demand, your heart rate and blood pressure increase or decrease as needed. But if blood pressure decreases too much and the brain receives insufficient oxygen, you faint.

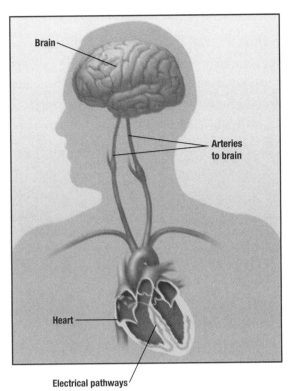

> Electrical signals that travel through conduction pathways in the heart tell the heart's chambers when to pump, sending a steady supply of oxygenated blood through two main arteries to the brain.

Your doctor may call your problem vasovagal syncope or orthostatic hypotension. Both of these are relatively benign conditions; you need not be too concerned about either one. They can be caused by:

- Strong feelings, such as anxiety or fear. This is the classic "movie-star swoon," and it really does happen. A nerve signal briefly changes heart rate and lowers blood pressure too much.
- Standing for too long. This can cause blood to pool in the legs, preventing the brain from receiving all the blood it needs.
- Sitting up from a reclining position or standing up too quickly. Blood pressure may not adjust rapidly enough to changes in posture and may temporarily drop too low. Certain medications, such as drugs used to treat hypertension, can also cause this problem.

Syncope that Stems from Heart Trouble

When a heart problem is the source of fainting spells, you need to take the situation seriously. Several types of heart trouble may cause syncope. For example, heart disease may be reducing the amount of oxygen and blood that reaches the brain. Your heart rate could be too slow or too fast, or a damaged heart valve might be decreasing blood flow. Any condition that keeps the heart from pumping enough blood can make your blood pressure drop too low and cause you to faint.

SYNCOPE FROM A SLOW HEART RATE

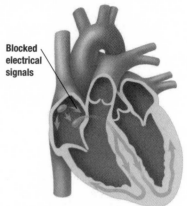

Blocked electrical signals

Sometimes the electrical signals that orchestrate the beating of the heart's four chambers may be slowed or blocked (heart block) as they travel the heart's electrical conduction pathways. When the heart rate slows, not enough blood gets pumped. The underlying cause of this disruption can be normal aging, scarred heart tissue, or damage from heart disease.

SYNCOPE FROM A FAST HEART RATE

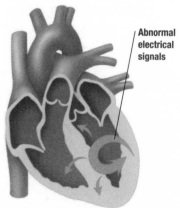

Abnormal electrical signals

Certain problems can make the heart race. After a heart attack, for instance, abnormal electrical signals can tell the heart's chambers to pump before they have a chance to fill with blood. As a consequence, less blood reaches the brain and other parts of the body. Illegal drugs, certain medications, heart disease, or an inherited condition can also cause this sort of accelerated heart rate.

SYNCOPE FROM A
HEART-VALVE PROBLEM

As explained in Chapter 1, valves in the heart open and close as the heart's chambers pump and relax, helping to keep blood moving in the right direction. But if a valve is hardened or scarred, it may not open or close fully. As a result, less blood is pumped through the heart to the brain and body.

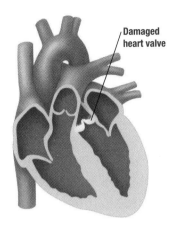

Damaged
heart valve

TREATING SYNCOPE

If you have syncope, your treatment options depend on what is causing it. You may be asked to:

- Adjust your diet or lifestyle to help avoid sudden drops in blood pressure.
- Take medication or adjust the dose of a medication you are already taking—such as a drug designed to control high blood pressure.
- Undergo a procedure or surgery to correct an underlying heart problem that may be causing you to faint.

Chapter 6 describes treatment options for syncope in more detail.

Palpitations: Disturbing Heartbeats

Your heart beats so steadily so often—the average person's heart pumps about 100,000 times a day—that you're usually not aware of it at all. Palpitations are a different story: You feel a strange pounding sensation in your chest or you have a disturbing consciousness of the pumping of your heart.

The standard accelerated *thump thump thump* that people experience during and after physical exertion is completely normal; it is nothing more than a sign of a healthy heart responding to extra work as it should. People with palpitations, by contrast, often describe a fluttering feeling—a sensation like that of a butterfly beating its wings inside their chest—or a thudding, skipped heartbeat, or a pounding in the chest or neck unrelated to any particular activity.

Palpitations are one of the symptoms most likely to send someone to the doctor seeking an evaluation for heart disease. But heart disease isn't always the culprit. In fact, the most common cause of palpitations is anxiety or tension. Smoking, drinking alcohol or beverages containing caffeine, or taking certain prescription medications such as thyroid pills, asthma drugs, and beta blockers (used to treat high blood pressure) can also create palpitations that have nothing to do with defects in the heart.

Palpitations and the Heart

Even when something about the heart itself is behind an episode of palpitations, heart disease may not be responsible. Older people with no underlying heart disease, for example, are more likely to experience occasional extra beats as a natural result of the aging process. But palpitations can be a sign of something seriously wrong with the heart, such as an arrhythmia, or abnormal heartbeat, that could potentially cause cardiac arrest. Anyone who experiences a series of rapid heartbeats while at rest—especially when the rapid beating lasts more than a few minutes—should get a medical evaluation as soon as possible.

An extremely rapid heart rate sometimes originates in the upper chambers, or atria, of the heart. These forms of arrhythmia are known as supraventricular tachycardia or paroxysmal atrial tachycardia and, while unpleasant, aren't a major cause for alarm. People with these conditions generally feel well except during the palpitations themselves, which usually don't last long, and there's little reason to suspect a dangerously advanced case of heart disease.

The most serious heart problem that causes palpitations is ventricular tachycardia, a life-threatening rapid heartbeat that occurs most often in people with well-established heart disease. As the name suggests, this form of rapid heartbeat originates in the ventricles, the lower chambers of the heart that do the heavy work of pumping blood to the lungs (right ventricle) and the rest of the body (left ventricle). In ventricular tachycardia, the ventricles quiver, or fibrillate, greatly reducing the heart's ability to pump blood out to the body. People with this condition often feel quite weak and short of breath as a result. Sometimes the heart is unable to pump any blood at all, in which case immediate medical help is required to prevent cardiac arrest, collapse, and sudden death. Defibrillators—the charged paddles long familiar from medical dramas and now appearing more frequently in public places such as airports and hotel lobbies—can restore the heartbeat of people who have collapsed from ventricular arrhythmias (see pages 261–262).

Claudication: Pain or Fatigue in the Limbs

About 9 million Americans—including 20 percent of those 70 and older—experience occasional claudication.

The buildup of plaque inside coronary arteries causes the most common form of heart disease, coronary artery disease (CAD). But atherosclerosis can also affect arteries in other parts of the body, in which case it is called peripheral arterial disease (PAD). When PAD occurs in the arteries of the legs, it creates a painful condition known as claudication, which means "limping." Here, severely restricted blood flow—or an outright blockage—produces cramping or aching in the buttocks, thighs, or calves after even a short walk. Climbing stairs or walking uphill tends to make claudication worse. Because the pain usually goes away when you stop exerting yourself but returns when you move again, medical practitioners often refer to it as intermittent claudication.

Sometimes also called "leg angina," claudication can be a tipoff that you have heart disease. How so? Because people with atherosclerosis in leg arteries are likely to have developed it in their coronary arteries as well. It can also mean that atherosclerosis has affected arteries in your brain, increasing your risk for a stroke.

If you experience claudication, undergo a medical evaluation at the earliest opportunity. You need to find out whether the athero-

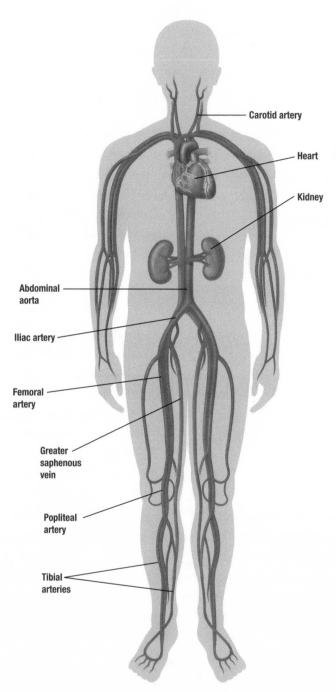

Carotid artery

Heart

Kidney

Abdominal aorta

Iliac artery

Femoral artery

Greater saphenous vein

Popliteal artery

Tibial arteries

> Peripheral arterial disease (PAD) usually occurs in the legs but can affect other blood vessels and organs such as the kidneys.

sclerosis responsible for your leg pain is also affecting your coronary arteries and putting you at risk for a heart attack.

Shortness of Breath (Dyspnea)

Everyone experiences shortness of breath occasionally—after walking up a flight of stairs, for example, or when carrying heavy luggage. But shortness of breath after a brief walk or while at rest is not normal. Indeed, shortness of breath constitutes one of the earliest and most common symptoms of heart disease.

Dyspnea—the medical term for abnormal shortness of breath—is defined as difficult, labored, or uncomfortable breathing. It may arise from conditions other than heart disease, such as emphysema, asthma, and other lung ailments. People who are overweight can easily become short of breath simply because of the extra weight they carry around. They may not yet have heart disease—but, of course, being overweight is one of heart disease's main risk factors.

Dyspnea that does trace to heart disease usually occurs when the heart's pumping action is weakened because narrowed coronary arteries cannot supply enough oxygen to the heart muscle or when the heart muscle has been damaged or its tissue has been thickened or thinned. In other cases, a narrowed or improperly opening heart valve may be keeping blood from flowing from one chamber to another. Dyspnea can also be a symptom of heart failure.

Consult a health care professional if you get winded by activities that previously didn't make you feel out of breath. An expert can help determine whether your shortness of breath is simply a matter of being out of shape or if it's a symptom of a serious health problem such as heart disease.

Fatigue

Fatigue accompanies many diseases, is a major symptom of depression, and typically afflicts the stressed and the sleep-deprived.

About 10 percent of people taking drugs to lower blood pressure experience fatigue.

Fatigue is also a common symptom of heart disease—specifically heart failure. Someone with heart failure typically begins the day with a normal energy level, then grows more and more tired. Over the course of the day, the heart muscle becomes continuously weaker as it increasingly loses its ability to pump enough blood and oxygen to sustain bodily functions.

Fatigue most likely stems from heart disease if it has developed over a short period of time. If that applies to you, consult your health care provider to see if the cause may be heart failure or some other heart problem.

People with heart disease may also feel fatigued because of medications they are taking. Other causes of fatigue include anemia and chronic diseases such as hypothyroidism, diabetes, and lung disease.

Edema

Edema, or swelling, occurs when fluid leaks from the bloodstream into surrounding tissues. Unlike fatigue, edema is almost always considered abnormal—and a probable indicator of disease. It's particularly common in heart disease and results from the heart's inability to function efficiently.

When the heart is not pumping at full strength—in the case of heart failure, for example—fluids in the bloodstream tend to back up rather than flowing through the circulatory system. This pooled fluid then leaks out of blood vessels into surrounding tissues, causing swelling or puffiness.

Some people retain as much as 10 pounds of fluid in their arms and legs from edema before heart failure becomes noticeable.

Making matters worse, the heart's inadequate pumping action eventually decreases the amount of blood flowing to the kidneys, which in turn causes the kidneys to fail to excrete excess liquids as urine. The extra fluid accumulates in the body and shows up as weight gain. Consider the possibility of edema if you notice any increase in your weight that is unrelated to your eating habits.

People often first notice edema in their feet and ankles, particularly after they've been standing or sitting for long periods. You should report any such signs of swelling to your health care provider. Edema that ascends to the thighs or the torso requires immediate medical attention.

Patient, Heed Thyself

If you experience one or more of the eight symptoms above—chest pain, angina, syncope, palpitations, claudication, dyspnea, fatigue, or edema—take them as possible warning signs of heart disease and get yourself evaluated. Treatments now available can halt heart disease in its tracks, prevent it from leading to heart attack and other serious consequences—and even reverse it.

When you describe your symptoms to your health care provider, he or she will question you about them and perform an exam. In most cases, you'll also undergo one or more diagnostic tests. These will help reveal how well (or not) your heart responds to stress and whether there is any damage to the heart muscle. Other tests can detect constriction of arteries and precisely where that narrowing is. All this information will ultimately assist your doctor in designing your treatment plan.

Health History & Physical Exam

A medical evaluation involves several steps. Your doctor will examine you, ask about your health history, and order blood tests.

- Medical history. Your doctor will ask about your health and the health of close relatives. He or she will ask about any angina symptoms and when they occur. Be sure to tell your doctor about any medications, herbs, or supplements you are taking.
- Physical exam. In addition to taking your blood pressure, your doctor will listen to your heartbeat and check how well blood flows through arteries.
- Blood tests. Your doctor will order tests for blood lipids such as cholesterol and triglycerides. You may also be tested for diabetes and other conditions that affect the heart.
- Follow-up tests. Depending on the results of your history and physical, your doctor may want to perform other tests to get a better idea of your heart health. Major tests that can reveal important information about your heart are described below.

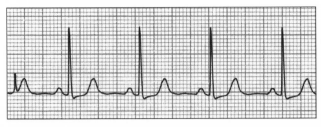

> During an ECG, your heart's electrical patterns are printed out on graph paper.

The Resting Electrocardiogram

The resting electrocardiogram (abbreviated as ECG or EKG) is one of the simplest and most common tests of heart health. It is often the first follow-up test to your medical history and physical exam.

During the ECG, you sit or lie down with leads (wires) attached to your arms, legs, and chest by small pads. The other ends are connected to a machine that detects electrical signals and shows them as a wave pattern on a screen. The test is completely painless.

The ECG records the heart's electrical patterns, which to the trained eye contain valuable information about how the heart is working. Among other things, the resting ECG can reveal a previously undetected heart attack or show whether a known attack has damaged your heart muscle.

The Echocardiogram

Like the resting ECG, an echocardiogram (or echo) is a safe, painless test of your heart. It uses high-frequency sound waves, commonly known as ultrasound, to show how well your heart muscle and valves are working and to gauge the size of your heart (an enlarged heart can be a sign of potentially serious problems). A transducer (a device that looks like a microphone) sends sound waves through your chest and bounces them off your heart. A computer then converts the sound waves into images that appear on a video screen.

The echo requires some preparation and thus may be done in a hospital or test center rather than a doctor's office. Expect it to take less than 45 minutes.

Before the test

When you schedule your echo test, be sure to mention what medications you take. Ask if it's okay to eat on the day of the test. Also ask if you need to arrive early to check in if you're taking the test at a hospital or other facility you're unfamiliar with. On the day of the test, wear a shirt, blouse, or sweater that you can remove easily.

During the echo

- Small pads (electrodes) are placed on your chest to monitor your heartbeat.
- A transducer coated with cool gel is moved firmly over your chest. It generates the sound waves that make images of your heart.
- You may be asked to breathe out and not breathe in for a few seconds; air in your lungs can affect the images.
- The images of your heart appear on a video monitor. They are recorded so your doctor can review them later.

A Doppler study may also be done during your echo. This ultrasound test uses the transducer to measure the direction and speed of blood flowing through your heart. During the Doppler study, you may hear a "whooshing" noise. This is the sound of your blood flowing.

After the echo

When the test is over, you can most likely eat and return to your normal routine. Find out if you should take any medication you were asked to skip before the test. During a future office visit, your doctor will discuss your test results with you.

Cardiac Nuclear Imaging

A sophisticated technique for detecting heart disease, cardiac nuclear imaging can locate areas of the heart muscle that are not getting enough blood. Your health care provider may want you to undergo a nuclear scan early in the effort to diagnose your heart problem, or you may have such a scan following a heart attack or other major cardiac event to evaluate the extent of any damage.

Don't let the word "nuclear" scare you: Nuclear imaging carries very little risk. Trace amounts of radioactive material (called radionuclides) that give off a tiny amount of radiation are injected into your bloodstream but stay in the body only briefly. Your radiation exposure during cardiac nuclear imaging is equivalent to the radiation from a bowel x-ray taken after swallowing barium.

A radiation-detecting device called a gamma camera monitors the progress of the "tracer" as it flows through the circulatory system. A computer processes the data, then displays it as still pictures of blood vessels and the heart. Some cameras are able to rotate around the patient, producing three-dimensional images of the heart known as tomograms.

There are two types of cardiac nuclear imaging: the MUGA scan and perfusion scanning.

MUGA SCAN
(EQUILIBRIUM RADIONUCLIDE ANGIOCARDIOGRAM)

The MUGA scan (MUltigated Graft Acquisition) is the more common of the two nuclear imaging techniques for assessing heart function—particularly the functioning of the left ventricle, the heart's main pumping chamber. A MUGA scan measures your heart's ejection fraction—the ability of your heart to pump blood with each beat.

A normal ejection fraction is around 60 percent. A low ejection fraction may indicate that blockages in the coronary arteries have weakened your left ventricle.

PERFUSION SCANNING

This type of cardiac nuclear imaging evaluates blood flow through the coronary arteries. Because this procedure employs the radioactive substance thallium, it is frequently called a thallium scan.

After flowing through the bloodstream from the point of injection, the thallium enters heart-muscle cells by way of the coronary

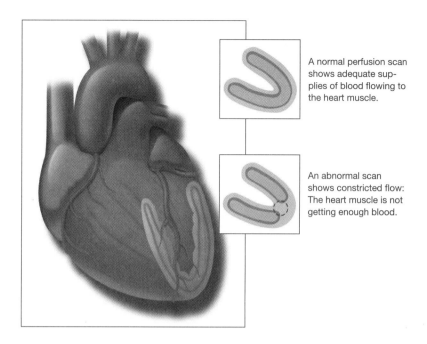

A normal perfusion scan shows adequate supplies of blood flowing to the heart muscle.

An abnormal scan shows constricted flow: The heart muscle is not getting enough blood.

arteries. During the scanning, images of the heart muscle show how well the muscle tissue is being "perfused" with blood—that is, how well blood is flowing into it.

You may undergo perfusion scanning while you engage in some form of exercise, then again after a rest period. By comparing how well your heart is perfused with blood under these two conditions, a cardiologist can assess the health of both your heart muscle and the arteries that supply it with blood.

The Exercise Test

The exercise test (also known as a stress ECG) is an ECG carried out while you walk on a treadmill or ride a stationary bike. In some cases, you will instead take a medication that stresses the heart without subjecting it to the more uncontrollable strain of actual physical activity.

The exercise test shows whether your coronary arteries can meet the increased demand for blood that occurs during exertion. It can also evaluate the cause of any chest pain you might be having and measure the strength of your heart. In addition, an exercise test can alert your doctor to the presence of previously undiagnosed heart-function abnormalities that may be triggered or aggravated by exercise.

If you've already had a heart attack, the exercise test can reveal how well you've progressed. Be aware that you may feel angina during an exercise test, even if you've never felt it before. You should also know that women are more likely than men to experience "false-positive" results from an exercise stress test, meaning that the test falsely indicates the presence of a heart abnormality.

Taking the exercise test

A typical exercise test takes about 30 minutes. You'll be told well in advance how to prepare for the test. Check to see how early you need to arrive. Discuss any questions you have with your doctor at least one day before.

When you schedule the test, be sure to mention *all* medications you take and ask if it is okay to take them as usual or if you need to skip a dose.

For three hours before the test:

- Don't eat.
- Don't drink. (If your doctor says you can take your medications, small sips of water are okay.)
- Don't smoke.
- Don't have any caffeine.

If you have diabetes, ask what you may eat before the test. Be aware that coffee, tea, chocolate, cola drinks, and some over-the-counter pain relievers may contain caffeine, which can skew the results. On the day of your exercise test, keep these tips in mind:

- Wear flat, comfortable walking shoes. Choose shoes that lace up or close with Velcro (rather than slip-ons). The shoes should have closed toes.
- Pick a shirt, blouse, or sweater that you can remove easily. You may be asked to undress from the waist up and put on a short hospital gown.

During your exercise test:

- Small electrodes with leads connecting them to a monitor are placed on your upper body. (The electrodes have an adhesive backing to help them attach to your skin.) A blood-pressure cuff is wrapped around your arm. Together these monitor your heartbeat and blood pressure during and after the test.
- You are shown how to use the treadmill or bike.
- You are then asked to exercise for several minutes. Expect the exercise to be easy at first. It will slowly get harder.
- Exercise as long as you can, or until you are asked to stop. You'll probably be encouraged to exercise until you are too tired to go on or until you experience symptoms such as angina or shortness of breath.

Report any symptoms

During the test, be sure to tell the health care provider if you feel any of the following:

- Chest, arm, or jaw discomfort
- Severe shortness of breath
- Fatigue
- Dizziness
- Leg cramps or soreness

After your exercise test

As soon as the test is over, you can eat and return to your normal routine. Ask your doctor about taking any medication that you were told to skip beforehand. Your doctor will discuss your test results with you. This might occur the day of the test or during a future office visit or phone call.

Cardiac Catheterization

A catheterization is any procedure in which a catheter (a long, thin, flexible tube) is inserted into the body. Cardiac catheterization means that the catheter is inserted into an artery in the groin or arm, then threaded through that artery and into your heart.

In a type of catheterization known as coronary angiography, contrast fluid is injected through the catheter once it's in place. As the contrast fluid fills the arteries, it makes the arteries stand out on x-ray images. An x-ray machine then takes pictures (angiograms) of the heart and coronary arteries. These images can reveal the presence of partial or total blockages of the coronary arteries.

Coronary angiography is often a follow-up to confirm the results of a less-invasive test (a resting ECG or echo, for example) that has identified a problem. The procedure can determine whether your coronary arteries are damaged, narrowed, or blocked. It can also tell how well your heart muscle and heart valves are functioning. The catheter can even measure blood pressure and oxygen levels inside the heart.

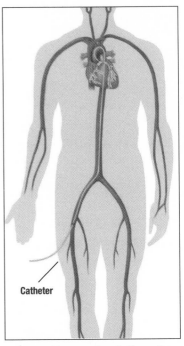

> Inserted into an artery in the groin, a catheter—a long, flexible tube—is gently pushed up the artery and into the heart.

Knowing what to expect during coronary angiography will help ease your mind. The procedure itself generally takes less than an hour. You will be awake the entire time and may be given medication to help you relax before the procedure begins. You shouldn't experience pain during the test, though you may feel the pressure of the moving catheter shortly after its insertion.

Before your catheterization, discuss the procedure's risks (see below) and any questions you have with your health care provider. Also tell your doctor if you're pregnant or have ever had an allergic reaction to iodine (found in shellfish). The night before the procedure, you may be asked not to eat or drink anything after midnight.

RISKS AND COMPLICATIONS OF CATHETERIZATION

There are risks associated with catheterization—some of them serious. In extremely rare cases, catheterization can cause a heart attack, stroke, or even death. Complications also occasionally necessitate emergency heart-bypass surgery. The more common types of problems that can result from catheterization include these:

- Bleeding or clotting
- Minor tearing of the artery lining
- Arrhythmia (abnormal heartbeat)
- Allergic reaction to the contrast dye, or related kidney problems

Electrophysiology Studies

Your heart rhythm is the speed and pattern of your heartbeat as the heart's chambers contract and relax. You may have already been diagnosed with a heart-rhythm problem such as an arrhythmia, or you may have symptoms that suggest one. Your doctor or cardiologist uses an electrophysiology study (EPS) to learn more. The EPS can reveal the source of any arrhythmia and help your doctor devise an effective treatment for it.

An EPS is a type of catheterization in which one or more electrode catheters—thin, soft, coated wires—are inserted through blood vessels into the chambers of the heart. The electrodes enable the cardiologist to closely monitor heart rhythm and the pumping action of each chamber. In some cases, an electrical current is sent through the electrode to trigger certain abnormal heart rhythms and allow the doctor to observe how the heart reacts. The doctor may even try various medications during the study to see if they help control an arrhythmia.

Before your electrophysiology study begins, you'll receive complete instructions on how to prepare for it. If you have any questions, ask your doctor. An EPS study usually takes one to two hours. You may be given a mild sedative to help you relax. Or the procedure may be performed under general anesthesia.

The day of the test, a nurse or EPS technician will wash and perhaps shave the area of skin on your groin, neck, or shoulder where the catheters will be inserted. You will also have a small intravenous catheter inserted in a vein in your arm for the delivery of any medications used during the EPS; these may include a sedative and any test medications that can help determine the best treatment.

Before the procedure:

- Tell your doctor about all prescription or over-the-counter medications you take. This includes herbs, supplements, and heart-rhythm medications. You may be told to stop taking some of them before the procedure.
- Don't eat or drink anything after midnight on the day before the procedure, unless told otherwise by your doctor.

INSERTING THE WIRES

Before inserting the catheters, the person conducting the test will numb the area with a local anesthetic. He or she then makes a small puncture in the blood vessel, inserts each catheter, and—with the help of x-ray monitors—gently threads them to your heart.

One or more of the following procedures may be done during the study:

- Electrical signals can be sent through the catheters to stimulate the heart and possibly induce an arrhythmia. The arrhythmia is monitored and its starting point is checked. If you're awake, you may feel your heartbeat changing or your heart racing from time to time.
- If arrhythmias are induced, they may be stopped with additional electrical signals that regulate, or pace, the heartbeat. Sometimes the heart is given an electric shock (defibrillation) to stop an arrhythmia.
- If an arrhythmia is diagnosed during EPS, your doctor may administer test medications to find the best drug for controlling the problem. Or, in a technique called catheter ablation, energy waves can be sent through a special electrode catheter to ablate, or destroy, the cells causing the rhythm problem.

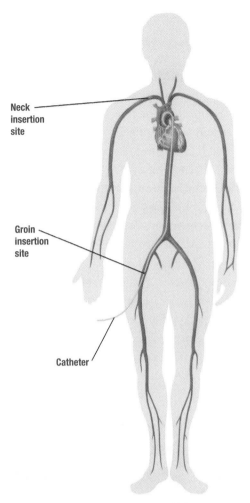

Neck insertion site

Groin insertion site

Catheter

> Possible insertion sites for the electrode catheter

UNDERSTANDING THE RISKS OF EPS

The risk of a complication from EPS is fairly low—less than 1 in 100. These rare complications can include:

- Bleeding
- Blood clots
- Collapsed lung
- Perforation of the heart muscle or a blood vessel
- Stroke or heart attack (very rare)
- Death (extremely rare)

The Calcium Scan

A calcium heart scan is a painless, noninvasive x-ray technique for detecting narrowing in your coronary arteries. It takes advantage of the fact that calcium (along with fat and cholesterol) is a major component of plaque—the fatty material that narrows arteries in the disease process of atherosclerosis.

The scan detects whether calcium is present and calculates how much is there—the patient's "calcium score." These scores can range from zero (no detectable plaque) to several thousand (extensive plaque). A number of studies have shown that patients' calcium scores can reliably predict their heart-attack risk.

Calcium scanners use one of two techniques: electron-beam computed tomography (EBCT), in which electron bursts are converted into x-rays, or helical (spiral) CT, in which an x-ray gun images the heart while spinning around the patient. Although most scanning centers use helical CT, EBCT—which takes about a minute—has a more extensively evaluated track record.

An EBCT scan starts with the patient lying on a table. As the table slides slowly into a scanner, a beam of electrons bounces off tungsten plates in the scanner and is converted into x-rays. The scanner captures 35 or more "slices" across the heart, each slice just 3 millimeters thick. Any calcium deposits stand out clearly. After the scan, a computer analyzes the size and density of all the calcium deposits that show up in the x-ray images and calculates a cumulative calcium score.

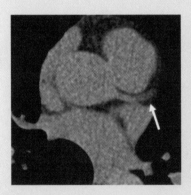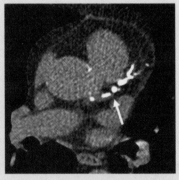

> EBCT can reveal fine detail in many structures of the heart. It can show portions of the coronary arteries and distinguish between those that are free of calcium deposits (arrow in left photo) and those that contain calcium deposits (arrow in right photo). Calcium deposits indicate the presence of atherosclerotic plaques and partial blockage of an artery. If calcium deposits are detected, aggressive use of therapies such as cholesterol-lowering drugs can prevent deposits from getting bigger and may even help to shrink them.
> *Images courtesy of John Rumberger, M.D.*

The Calcium Scan *continued*

A Controversial Test

Despite its reliability in assessing heart-attack risk, calcium heart scanning has become embroiled in the debate over the value of "whole body scanning" now being offered at imaging centers around the United States. These centers also provide scans of only the heart.

Proponents say that heart scans can detect heart disease at an early stage, allowing patients and their doctors to take steps that keep the disease from worsening. Critics contend that scanning the hearts of healthy people can cause harm if insignificant findings lead to invasive and possibly risky tests such as coronary angiography or treatments such as bypass surgery. If you are contemplating a calcium heart scan, first discuss the pros and cons with your health care provider.

When your EPS is over, you'll be taken to a recovery room, where you'll need to remain lying down for about four hours. To prevent bleeding, you will be asked not to move your leg if the catheter was inserted in your groin. During this time, your condition will be closely monitored. The medications given to you during the procedure may make you feel groggy and forgetful for a few hours. This is common and is nothing to worry about.

You may be able to go home the day of your EPS, or you may have to stay in the hospital overnight. When it's time to go, have an adult family member or friend drive you. You'll likely be able to return to your normal routine within a few days.

Your doctor will discuss your EPS results with you. The study, along with other test results, may provide enough information for your doctor to develop a treatment plan. Once you return home, call your doctor if you notice any of the following:

- Increased bruising or swelling
- Increased bleeding or pain at the insertion site
- Shortness of breath or chest pain
- A fever of more than 101° F (38.3° C)
- Dizziness, weakness, or unusual tiredness
- Worsening symptoms of your heart-rhythm problem

Living Well with 5
Heart Disease

Y OU MAY HAVE HAD bypass surgery or angioplasty, or you may be taking medication to modify a risk factor for heart disease—a diuretic for high blood pressure, for example. As essential as these medical interventions often are, they should never be the whole story. This chapter describes what you can do on your own to manage your heart disease and assess the risk factors it presents.

Whether you have a diagnosed case of heart disease or you are still coping only with risk factors, *now* is the time to make changes in your lifestyle to protect your arteries and help prevent a heart attack or stroke. Most people at risk can do something about the way they live—exercising more, for example, or switching to a low-fat diet—that will make a big difference.

Improving Heart Health with Exercise

To preserve your health, you must get (and stay) physically active. People who remain on the move have fewer heart attacks than those who live a more sedentary lifestyle. One way to start becoming more active is to turn aspects of your everyday routine into more physical undertakings: Climb the stairs rather than riding the elevator, for example, or park at the far end of the lot and walk briskly to the store. Best of all, you can engage in a formal exercise program.

If you need encouragement, learning more about the rewards of becoming active may help you get started. But the primary motivation must be the desire for a better life for yourself—a goal you can achieve by making exercise part of your daily regimen.

Overcome Your Obstacles

Adding exercise to an already-hectic life may seem overly ambitious—and that feeling may be just one of the hurdles you face. Remember that you can start as gradually as you need to, and that you will very likely find exercise an enjoyable part of your life. If you've tried before and stopped, look for a new activity you might like more.

If you still find yourself resistant to getting started, ask yourself why. Write your answers in the box below; then, beside each answer, list ways you can vault that particular obstacle.

Even if you have physical limitations, some form of exercise is usually feasible. Swimming or walking in a pool, for example, can be helpful for those with painful joints.

My Hurdles Are:	Ways I Can Overcome My Hurdles:
_____	_____
_____	_____
_____	_____
_____	_____

Exercise Feels Good

In addition to being beneficial for your body, exercise can help you enjoy a better life. People who have started exercising and have kept it up say they feel:

- Better about themselves.
- More upbeat about life.
- More energetic.
- More relaxed.
- Less stressed.
- Able to sleep better.

It's Good for You, Too

Exercising regularly offers many health benefits. It can help you:

- By allowing your heart to work less hard.
- Lower your blood pressure to help prevent a stroke or heart attack.

- Improve your heart function.
- Reach and maintain a healthy weight.
- Make your muscles stronger and more limber so you can stay active.
- Prevent falls and fractures by slowing the loss of bone mass from osteoporosis.
- Manage stress better.

Before Getting Started

Before you launch into a formal exercise program, your health care provider may advise you to have an exercise test, which measures how your body responds to exercise. You will most likely be asked to walk on a treadmill or ride an exercise bike for at least several minutes; you may also undergo other special cardiac tests. After gauging the results, your practitioner can work with you to devise a safe, effective exercise program.

Questions about exercise?

Talk with your health care provider before starting an exercise program. Be sure to bring up all of your concerns and questions. Below are some questions that people with heart disease often ask about exercise:

- *Is an exercise program safe for my heart?*
  Exercise can help your heart in many ways. If you have safety concerns, ask your health care provider whether you should take an exercise stress test first.
- *How will I know my exercise program is helping me?*
  You should be able to exercise longer with less effort during each session. Your heart rate may also be lower than it used to be, both at rest and when you're exercising.
- *What should I do if my heart beats unusually fast or slow or irregularly during exercise? What if I feel pain or discomfort in my chest, neck, back, or arms (angina)? What if I have unusual shortness of breath?*
  Stop exercising right away and call your health care provider.

Ensuring Safety & Comfort

If you feel safe and comfortable while exercising, you are more likely to enjoy your workouts—and more likely to maintain your exercise program. Following the guidelines below can help ensure your safety and comfort. If you have any questions, be sure to ask your health care provider.

Exercising safely

Following a few guidelines can help you exercise safely. Exercise indoors on particularly hot, cold, humid, or windy days, or when there are warnings about poor air quality. If you don't go to a gym, you can get indoor exercise at a shopping mall or community center. Drink plenty of water before and after exercise, and take frequent hydration breaks during exercise. If you take medication for angina, always carry it with you.

Dressing right for exercise

When dressing for exercise, it's best to wear loose-fitting clothes. Put on layers so you can take something off if you get too hot. Always wear shoes that fit well and are designed for exercise. If you exercise outside, wear a hat when it's cold to retain more of your body heat. Protect your eyes and skin from the sun with a wide-brimmed hat or visor and sunscreen.

Easing into Exercise

You may have been active before. Or perhaps this is the first time you've begun an exercise program. Either way, ease into your routine. Remember that you needn't become a hard-core hardbody in order to get fit. Set and achieve small goals, then build on those successes.

How much exercise is enough? To address that question, the U.S. government issued new dietary and exercise guidelines in 2005. The key recommendation is to "engage in regular physical activity and reduce sedentary activities to promote health, psychological well-being, and a healthy body weight." The guidelines make some more specific recommendations as well:

If You Have Diabetes

- Talk with your health care provider before starting any exercise program.
- Eat one to two hours before exercise. Carry glucose tablets or a snack. If symptoms of low blood sugar appear, take the tablets or eat the snack.
- Carry a medical ID card or wear a medical alert bracelet clearly indicating you have diabetes.
- Check your blood sugar before and after exercise. Don't exercise if your blood sugar is above 240.
- Wear shoes that fit well and seamless cotton socks.
- After exercise, check your feet for any sores, blisters, or spots that may be red or tender.

- To reduce the risk of chronic disease in adulthood: Engage in at least 30 minutes of moderate-intensity physical activity, above your usual activity, at work or home on most days of the week. For most people, greater health benefits can be obtained by engaging in physical activity of more vigorous intensity or longer duration.
- To manage body weight and prevent gradual, unhealthy weight gain in adulthood: Engage in about 60 minutes of moderate to vigorous activity on most days of the week. To complement these workouts, do not exceed daily caloric-intake requirements (1800 for women, 2200 for men).
- To sustain weight loss in adulthood: Participate in at least 60 to 90 minutes of daily moderate-intensity physical activity without exceeding caloric-intake requirements. Some people may need to consult with a health care provider before participating in this level of activity.

To summarize: Based on your goals, you should aim to accomplish 30 to 90 minutes of brisk exercise on most days—or, ideally, on every day—of the week. That objective may lie several stages away for you at this point. But if you take things one step at a time, you're bound to succeed.

Besides starting an exercise program, try being more active in general throughout the day. Walk as much as you can on errands. Take on more household tasks or yardwork. Rather than chatting on the phone, go out for a walk with a friend. Instead of watching TV, visit a local park or go dancing.

A daily habit not to break

You will reap the greatest rewards if you exercise every day, preferably for 60 to 90 minutes. You need not complete your entire routine at once. If it's more convenient, the same results can be achieved with three smaller workouts interspersed through the day.

The right kind of exercise

All exercise is good, but the right kind of exercise can improve how your heart functions. Whatever the regimen, you need to move at a brisk pace so your heart beats faster, you breathe harder, and (in some cases) you break a sweat. The right kind of exercise is also the type that works best with your lifestyle, that is safe, fun, and comfortable for you—and that fits your schedule and budget.

Picking your best options

With your health care provider's advice, you may have a fairly wide range of exercise choices. Swimming, walking, jogging, and riding a bike can all improve heart health. So can fitness classes, exercise videos, and many other forms of aerobic activity. You have to judge what works best for you. One good option is to change activities every once in a while, or even from day to day. You may need to experiment a bit to find the right formula that will keep your interest up—and keep you at it.

Why walking works

Walking is easy. Walking is fun. And you don't need any special equipment—just a pair of sturdy, well-fitting walking shoes. It can

Sample Walking Program										
Week	1	2	3	4	5	6	7	8	9	10
Minutes walking	10	10	15	15	20	20	25	25	30	30
Walks per week	3–4	3–4	3–4	4–5	4–5	4–5	5–6	5–6	6–7	6–7

> Follow this walking program for the first 10 weeks, or walk as instructed by your health care provider. To track your progress and see how much you've achieved, start writing in the exercise log on page 104.

also be social: Try walking with friends, neighbors, family members, a social group, your bowling team—whomever!

Set attainable goals: Walking 10 minutes a day is a reasonable target for those just starting out. Then slowly build up to 30 to 90 minutes a day. If you choose walking, you can begin with the program outlined above. Or you might ask your health care provider for advice.

If your levels of food consumption and other physical activities stay the same, you'll shed a pound of fat for every 35 miles you walk.

The Elements of Exertion

Regardless of your choice of activity, make it part of a regular routine. Exercise on as many days as you can—every day, if possible. Ideally your routine will include a warm-up period, some moderate-intensity (brisk) exercise, and a cool-down session. Add muscle-strengthening exercises to your aerobic routine two or three times a week.

Strengthen Your Muscles

Besides making your muscles stronger, strength exercises can improve your overall heart health. Stronger muscles help keep your heart rate and blood pressure from rising too much when you do lifting tasks, such as carrying groceries, thus minimizing the stress on your heart. Do strength exercises at the end of your routine, right before you stretch.

Pace yourself

Moving briskly is the goal, but don't overdo it. To strike the right balance, learn to judge how hard you are exercising. Pace yourself by checking your pulse (heart rate) or by using the talk test (see below), or by doing both. Ask your health care provider which method is best for you.

USE THE TALK TEST

The talk test can help you find out how hard you're exercising. Try talking during moderate-intensity exercise. You should be able to carry on a conversation without slowing down your exercise. If you are too out of breath to talk comfortably, you're likely exercising too hard. Slow down and find a pace that lets you talk with less effort.

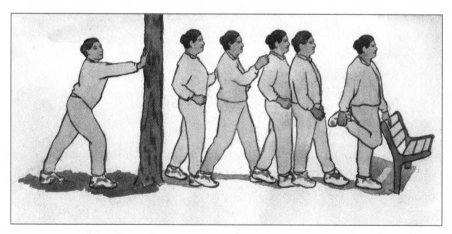

> **Start with a Warm-Up**
Start with a 10- to 15-minute warm-up that includes both your chosen exercise and some stretches. Warming up raises your heart rate slowly and loosens your muscles. Exercise at a slow pace for at least five minutes. Then stretch (see pages 10 and 11) for at least five minutes.

> **Get Your Heart Going**
Moderate-intensity exercise does the most good for your heart. Exercise at a brisk pace. At first, 10 minutes may be all you can do. In time you should be able to exercise at least 30 minutes a day. After this part of your routine, be sure to cool down.

> **Cool Down and Stretch**
Cooling down lowers your heart rate and blood pressure gradually. This keeps you from getting lightheaded and helps you recover from exercise. Do your chosen exercise at a very slow pace for five to seven minutes. Then stretch for five to seven minutes.

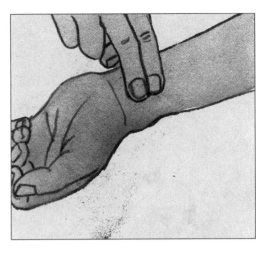

> Check your pulse on the inside of the wrist, below the base of the thumb.

TAKE YOUR PULSE

Your pulse reveals how fast your heart is beating, so monitoring it is a good way to rate your effort. Find out from your health care provider what your heart rate should be at rest and during exercise, then check your pulse before, during, and after exercise. Gently press your index and middle fingers against the inside of your wrist. Count the number of beats you feel for 10 seconds, then multiply that number by six to calculate beats per minute. If you're above or below your target pulse, adjust the intensity of your workout.

Stretching your muscles

Stretching your muscles loosens them up and can help protect them from injury. During the warm-up, stretching prepares your muscles for exercise. As you cool down, stretching lengthens and relaxes them. Try to do most or all of the stretches illustrated below each time you exercise. When you stretch one arm or leg, always repeat that stretch with the other arm or leg. If you've recently had heart surgery, talk with your health care provider about which of these stretches (or other ones) you should do.

- Have chest pain.
- Feel burning, tightness, pressure, or heaviness in your chest, neck, shoulders, back, or arms.
- Have unusual shortness of breath.
- Have a pulse that is much faster or slower than expected.
- Feel dizzy or lightheaded.
- Have increased joint pain.
- Have increased muscle pain.

Don't exercise on days when you are ill or have forgotten to take any prescription medication.

Head Tilt

1. Sit or stand with your shoulders relaxed.
2. Slowly lower your chin until you feel a stretch in the back of your neck.

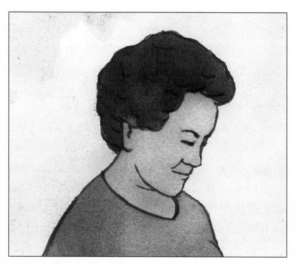

> Head Tilt

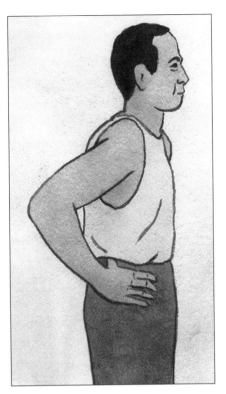

> Shoulder Roll

Shoulder Roll

1. Stand with your shoulders relaxed.
2. Put your hands on your hips.
3. Slowly roll your shoulders forward four to six times.
4. Roll your shoulders backward four to six times.

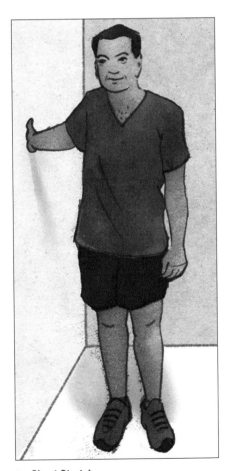

> Chest Stretch

Chest Stretch

1. Stand with your right arm and side next to a wall.
2. Place your right hand on the wall behind you at chest level with your arm outstretched.
3. Slowly turn your upper body away from the wall. Feel the stretch in your chest and right arm.
4. Repeat the stretch, this time with your left arm and side next to the wall.

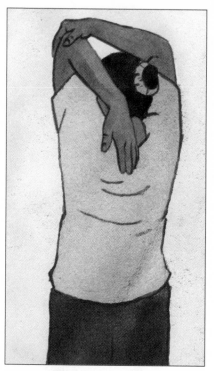

> Triceps Stretch

Triceps Stretch

1. Sit or stand.
2. With your left arm and hand, reach for your shoulder blades.
3. Use your right hand to press your left elbow downward. Feel the stretch in the back of your left upper arm (triceps).
4. Repeat the stretch, this time reaching for your shoulder blades with your right arm and hand.

Calf Stretch

1. Stand facing a wall. Put both hands on the wall.
2. Step back with your left foot. Keep your toes pointed forward and your right knee slightly bent.
3. Lean into the wall, keeping your left heel on the floor. Feel the stretch in the back of your lower leg (calf).
4. Repeat for the other calf by stepping back with your right foot.

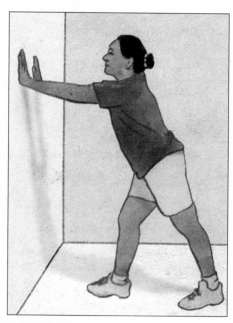

> Calf Stretch

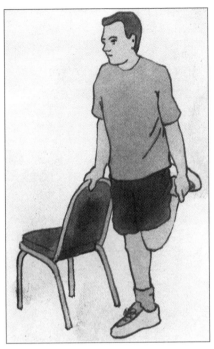

> Quadriceps Stretch

Quadriceps Stretch

1. Stand beside a sturdy chair. Hold the back of the chair with your right hand for balance.
2. With your left hand, grasp the top of your left foot or ankle and pull your left leg upward so that it bends at the knee. Keep your knee pointed toward the floor. Feel the stretch in the front of your thigh (quadriceps).
3. Repeat the sequence with your right foot to stretch the quadriceps in your other leg.

Back Stretch

1. Lie on your back on a mat with your legs extended.
2. Raise one knee toward your chest and grasp your leg behind the bent knee. (You can keep the other knee slightly bent.) Feel the stretch in your lower back, buttocks, and the back of your thigh.
3. Repeat with your other leg.

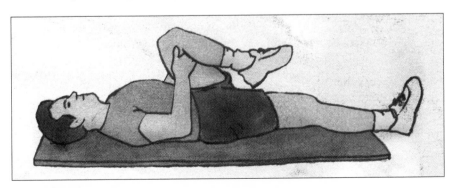

> Back Stretch

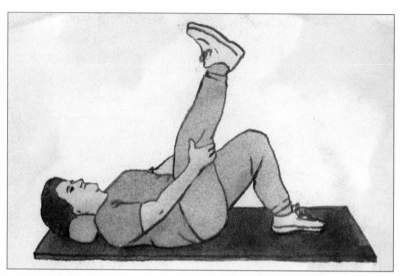

> Hamstring Stretch

Hamstring Stretch

1. Lie on your back on a mat with your knees bent and your feet flat.
2. Using both hands, slowly raise one knee toward your chest.
3. Grasp your calf or your thigh. Slowly straighten your raised leg until you feel a stretch in the back of your thigh (hamstring).
4. Repeat to stretch the hamstring in your other leg.

HELPFUL HINTS FOR STRETCHING

- Stay relaxed and breathe normally when you stretch. Don't hold your breath.
- Hold each stretch (except the shoulder rolls) for 10 to 20 seconds.
- When stretching, you should feel a gentle pull on the muscles being exercised. Avoid jerking movements. If you feel any pain, stop stretching.

Building up strength

Strength exercises do more than make your muscles stronger and lessen the stress on your heart. They also help control your weight and keep your bones strong. Do the exercises below two or three times a week, right before you stretch. Repeat each exercise 10 to 15 times. Before trying any of these exercises, however, talk with your health care provider. Make sure to ask which hand weights are right for you.

Chest Press

1. Lie on a bench or mat with your knees bent and your feet flat. With your arms bent, hold a weight in each hand.
2. Exhale and slowly press the weights toward the ceiling until your arms are almost straight.
3. Inhale and slowly lower the weights to their starting position.

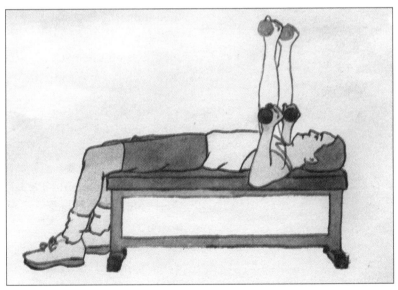

> Chest Press

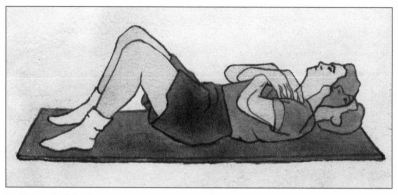

> Abdominal Curl

Abdominal Curl

1. Lie on your back on a mat with your knees bent and your feet flat. Look up at the ceiling. Cross your arms over your chest.
2. Contract your stomach (abdominal) muscles. Exhale and slowly lift your head and shoulders off the mat.
3. Inhale. Slowly return to the starting position.

Shoulder Press

1. Stand while holding a weight in each hand at shoulder level. Your palms should face forward.
2. Exhale and slowly press the weights toward the ceiling until your arms are almost straight.
3. Inhale and slowly lower the weights to shoulder level.

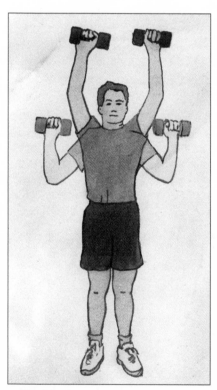

> Shoulder Press

Biceps Curl

1. Stand with a weight in each hand. Keep your arms straight, palms facing forward.
2. Exhale and slowly bend your arms, lifting the weights to shoulder level.
3. Inhale and slowly lower the weights to their starting position.

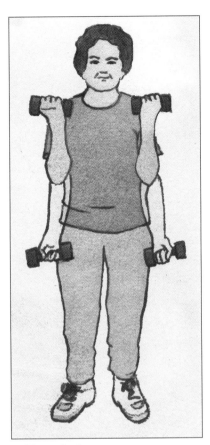

> Biceps Curl

Tracking your progress

Once you've started exercising routinely, track your progress. You can do this by writing in an exercise log such as the one provided on page 104. Monitoring the progress you've made in your program can help keep you motivated. It can also help you spot areas where you may need to make adjustments.

USING YOUR EXERCISE LOG

Use your exercise log daily. Even noting that you didn't exercise—and why you didn't—can help you keep tabs on your progress. Complete each part of the log to learn what feels right for you, and what doesn't. Exercising too hard one day, for instance, may leave

Exercise Log

Begin tracking your progress in this exercise log. When it is full, start your own log in a calendar or notebook.

Date	Time	Activity	Goal	Minutes	Comments
5/18	9 a.m.	Walking	10 minutes	10	Felt energized

you feeling too tired to work out the next. Finally, be sure to review your entire exercise log now and then to see how far you've come.

Reward Yourself!

You'll soon start reaping the benefits of exercise. You may notice your weight dropping or, during a checkup, you may learn that your blood pressure has improved. Or you may simply feel better.

A healthier you is a reward in itself, but you should also treat yourself more overtly when you reach a certain goal or receive an improved health report. Think of rewarding your own efforts as a behavioral incentive to keep up the good work. Such inducements can be anything you have put off enjoying until you achieve a specific goal, but take care to avoid "backsliding" treats: an unhealthy snack you've given up, for example, or a calorie-laden meal. To stay the course, consider some of these alternatives:

- Visit an art museum with friends.
- Go bowling or fishing.
- Take an active vacation, such as a trip to a national park where you can walk and go hiking.
- Shop for new books or music.
- Buy a new outfit—a necessity, perhaps, for your leaner physique!

Staying Fit for Life

Exercise is one of the best things you can do for yourself every day. But it isn't always easy to maintain your routine. If you get out of the habit of exercising regularly, remind yourself that exercise is your ticket to a healthy future. Follow the advice below to stick to your program and stay fit for life.

You might miss a workout—or even several days of exercise—once in a while, but this doesn't mean you've failed. If you return to your routine in a few days, you'll lose none of the health benefits you've already achieved. These tips may help you keep exercising:

- To make exercise a habit, do your routine at the same time each day. You may want to try exercising first thing in the morning, before the day's schedule fills up.
- When you're busy, plan ahead for your exercise and make room for workout sessions in your schedule.
- If you feel tired or lazy before a workout, allow yourself to go light. You may find yourself gaining energy as the workout progresses.
- If you're often sore or tired after a workout, you may be exercising too hard. Try doing lighter workouts for a few days.
- Make exercise fun. Switch from one type of exercise to another. Do your routine with a friend or listen to music while you exercise. Some people find that certain music makes them exercise more vigorously.

It's Your Call

For fitness classes or a place to exercise, call a local hospital and ask about any cardiac-rehabilitation programs in your area. Look into joining a local fitness club or gym, or try a recreation center or community college. The Appendix of this book contains additional suggestions on how to locate a program or design one yourself.

Heart-Healthy Eating

What you eat makes a big difference to your heart. Some foods improve heart health. Others contain substances that have been linked to high blood pressure and heart disease. Unfortunately, many of us grew up on diets that trained us to prefer foods more likely to harm our hearts—and our overall health.

But there is good news, too: You can eat healthfully for your heart and still enjoy the foods you like. This section provides some helpful hints for trimming the three main dietary culprits—fat, cholesterol, and salt—without losing flavor or sacrificing the pleasures of dining out.

What Are Your Risks?

Chapter 3 discussed some of the important conditions known to put you at a higher risk for heart disease or a heart attack. The list included:

- High cholesterol
- High blood pressure (hypertension)
- Excess weight
- Diabetes (high blood sugar)
- Smoking

Any one of these risk factors can increase your odds of developing a heart problem, but modifying one or more of them can significantly reduce your chance of developing heart disease or suffering a heart attack. And you can mitigate—or even eliminate—these risk factors by changing the way you eat.

Even if heart disease runs in your family, cutting down on fat, cholesterol, and salt lowers your risk of the illness. Losing excess weight cuts your risk as well. Not only that, but eating right and losing excess weight helps control diabetes and prevents damage to blood vessels.

What Is a Healthy Diet?

The American Heart Association and the National Cholesterol Education Program have set guidelines for a healthy diet. Each day, your diet should include:

- 30 percent or less of total calories from fat
- No more than 7 to 10 percent of total calories from saturated fat
- Less than 200 to 300 milligrams (mg) of cholesterol
- No more than 2,400 mg of sodium

Learning how to eat within these guidelines may take a little time. Your health care provider and written sources such as this book can help. But the choice to eat for a healthier heart is yours.

What Are You Doing Now?

You may already be doing smart things for your heart. Ask yourself these questions:

- Do I eat at least five servings of fruits and vegetables a day?
- Do I choose lean cuts of meat and low-fat or nonfat dairy foods?
- Do I compare food labels for fat, cholesterol, and sodium when I shop?
- Do I eat mostly fresh foods?
- Do I get some physical activity on most days?

If you answered any of these questions with a "Yes," pat yourself on the back: You are taking steps toward a healthier heart. But what about your "No" answers? Do you see ways you might make small changes? Read on for some practical ideas on how to get started.

A healthy diet:

• lowers your risk for heart disease, heart attack, and stroke.

• lowers your risk for colon cancer, breast cancer, and other cancers.

• helps you maintain a healthy weight. (Your health care provider can help you determine the ideal weight for you.)

• gives you more energy.

Size & Number Matter

The amount in a serving depends on the type of food and its group. The number of servings you should eat from each food group, in turn, hinges on your weight and activity level. Your health care provider can help you set the number of servings you need from each group. The chart on page 109 presents examples of five serving sizes.

How much is a serving?

Serving sizes are often expressed in units of cups or ounces, but you can't always make such precise measurements. Instead, you can use your own hand as a rough guide. A fist is approximately one cup.

WAYS TO AVOID EATING TOO MUCH

• Use smaller plates. It's a simple way to make less food look like more.

• Serve yourself smaller portions; don't go back for seconds.

• Eat slowly. It takes time for your body to register that you're full. If you eat too quickly, you'll wind up eating more than you need.

• Don't clean your plate out of habit. You can always put leftovers in the refrigerator.

• Never eat standing up or while watching TV.

• Don't finish food that others leave.

Eating the Right Size and Number of Servings

Food Group	Equivalents	Amount Per Day*	My Amount Per Day
Grains	1 ounce is equal to 1 slice bread 1 cup dry cereal ½ cup cooked rice, pasta, or cereal	6 ounces a day (at least 3 ounces should be whole grains)	
Vegetables	½ cup is equal to ½ cup raw or cooked vegetables 1 cup raw leafy greens ½ cup vegetable juice	2½ cups a day	
Fruits	½ cup is equal to 1 medium piece fresh fruit ½ cup fresh, frozen, or canned fruit ¼ cup dried fruit	2 cups a day	
Oils	1 teaspoon is equal to 1 teaspoon vegetable oil Oil is hidden in other foods. You probably get plenty in the food you eat.	6 teaspoons a day	
Milk	1 cup is equal to 1 cup low-fat or fat-free milk or yogurt 1½ ounces natural cheese 2 ounces processed cheese	3 cups a day	
Meat and Beans	1 ounce is equal to 1 ounce meat, fish, or poultry 1 egg 1 tbsp. peanut butter ¼ cup tofu	5½ ounces a day	

*Based on a 2,000-calorie diet

1 teaspoon The tip of the thumb	1 tablespoon A thumb (from the knuckle)	½ cup A cupped hand	1 cup A fist	2 to 3 ounces A small palm
For example: butter on a roll	For example: salad dressing	For example: fruits	For example: brown rice	For example: lean chicken

- When you dine out, ask for a take-home bag. Instead of overeating tonight, enjoy the food again tomorrow. You can even ask for a take-home bag before you begin eating, then immediately put half the meal inside it.

Using the Food Pyramid

The FDA's new Food Guide Pyramid, shown opposite, gives a detailed picture of a healthy diet. It can help you choose the right kinds of foods and the right amounts to eat. The larger the section of the pyramid, the more servings of those foods you should eat. Here are some other rough guidelines:

- Limit your intake of foods in the smaller sections.
- Limit the fat and oil you add to foods.
- Choose olive oil, canola oil, safflower oil, sunflower oil, or liquid margarine. Use only small amounts.

Milk, Yogurt, and Cheese: ½ to 8 g of fat in a serving
- Choose nonfat or low-fat milk or low-fat or nonfat buttermilk.
- Try nonfat yogurt and low-fat or nonfat cottage cheese.
- Look for reduced-fat or nonfat cheese.

Bread, Cereal, Rice, and Pasta: 1 g of fat in a serving
- Build your meals around these foods.
- Choose oatmeal and whole-grain bread, pasta, and dry cereal.
- Try brown rice, corn tortillas, couscous, millet, or kasha.

Vegetables: No fat in most servings
- Eat at least three servings a day.
- Choose dark-green, leafy vegetables; deep-yellow vegetables; and starchy vegetables such as potatoes.

Meat, Poultry, Fish, Beans, Eggs, and Nuts: 3 to 8 g of fat in a serving
- Choose fish, dried beans, tofu, and chicken or turkey breast most often.
- Look for red meat with little or no visible fat.

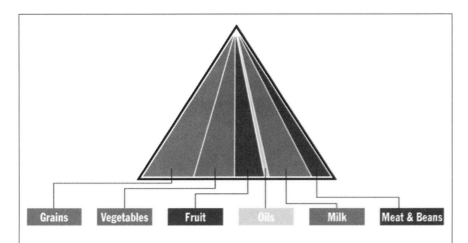

Grains

- At least half the grains you eat should be whole grains. Look for foods that list a whole grain (such as whole wheat or whole rolled oats) as the first ingredient.
- Foods made with whole grains, such as barley soup, are good choices.

Vegetables

- All vegetables are high in nutrients. The color of the skin tells you what's inside. If you eat plenty of different colored vegetables, you'll get a variety of nutrients.
- Good choices include: dark green vegetables (spinach, collard greens, broccoli); bright red and orange vegetables (carrots, red bell peppers, tomatoes); starchy vegetables (potatoes, squash).

Fruit

- Most of your fruit should come from whole sources. Try any fruit that's fresh, frozen, or canned in its own juice (no sugar added).
- Juice is high in calories and has less fiber than whole fruit. If you drink juice, make it 100% fruit juice (no sugar added).

Oils

- Oils are fats that are liquid at room temperature. This group includes oils you cook with, plus foods that are mostly oil, such as mayonnaise and salad dressing.
- You need some oils and fats to stay healthy. Too much, by contrast, leads to weight gain and increased heart-disease risk.

Milk

- This group includes milk as well as foods made from milk that are also high in calcium (such as cheese, cottage cheese, and yogurt).
- Choose low-fat or nonfat milk products.
- If you're allergic to milk, get calcium from leafy greens and from calcium-fortified foods such as orange juice and soy products.

Meat & Beans

- This group includes foods high in protein (meat, poultry, fish, soy products, beans, nuts, seeds, and eggs). Try to get protein from a variety of sources.
- Look for meat with little or no visible fat. Before cooking, trim away all the fat you can see.

Fruit: No fat in most servings

- Eat at least two servings a day. Include them in meals or treat them as snacks.
- Eat fresh fruits most often. Make sure fruit juice is 100 percent fruit.

What's in a Label?

Reading food labels is one of the best ways to ensure you are eating for a healthier heart. The labels on canned, packaged, and frozen foods give useful information about the nutritional content of those products. Comparing the labels can help you choose foods that are low in fat, cholesterol, and calories.

Look for the box on the label that says "Nutrition Facts." Then look at the numbers for each of the items highlighted in the sample nutrition box on page 113.

Serving size

This is the amount of food in a single serving. Ask yourself if this is the amount you will eat. If you eat more than one serving (two cookies, in this example), you'll get more of everything on the label—including fat, cholesterol, and calories.

Total fat

This number tells you how many grams (g) of fat a single serving contains. Choose foods with the lowest numbers for total fat. "Total fat" includes monounsaturated, unsaturated, and saturated fats, as well as trans fats.

Saturated fat

This number reveals how many grams of saturated fat are in a serving. Because saturated fat raises the level of low-density lipoprotein (LDL, or "bad" cholesterol) in your blood, look for foods with little or no saturated fat.

Trans fat

This number indicates how many grams of trans fat are in one serving. Trans fats are formed through a process that changes liquid fats into solid fats, and—like saturated fats—they increase levels of LDL cholesterol in the blood. Trans fats are also harmful because they lower blood levels of HDL ("good" cholesterol). So try to choose foods containing little or no trans fat.

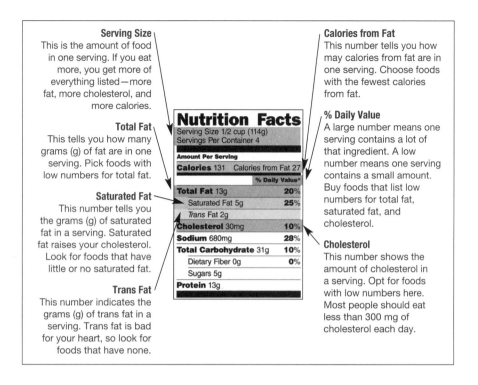

Serving Size
This is the amount of food in one serving. If you eat more, you get more of everything listed—more fat, more cholesterol, and more calories.

Total Fat
This tells you how many grams (g) of fat are in one serving. Pick foods with low numbers for total fat.

Saturated Fat
This number tells you the grams (g) of saturated fat in a serving. Saturated fat raises your cholesterol. Look for foods that have little or no saturated fat.

Trans Fat
This number indicates the grams (g) of trans fat in a serving. Trans fat is bad for your heart, so look for foods that have none.

Calories from Fat
This number tells you how may calories from fat are in one serving. Choose foods with the fewest calories from fat.

% Daily Value
A large number means one serving contains a lot of that ingredient. A low number means one serving contains a small amount. Buy foods that list low numbers for total fat, saturated fat, and cholesterol.

Cholesterol
This number shows the amount of cholesterol in a serving. Opt for foods with low numbers here. Most people should eat less than 300 mg of cholesterol each day.

Nutrition Facts
Serving Size 1/2 cup (114g)
Servings Per Container 4

Amount Per Serving

Calories 131   Calories from Fat 27

% Daily Value*

Total Fat 13g   20%
    Saturated Fat 5g   25%
    Trans Fat 2g
Cholesterol 30mg   10%
Sodium 680mg   28%
Total Carbohydrate 31g   10%
    Dietary Fiber 0g   0%
    Sugars 5g
Protein 13g

Calories from fat

Look at calories and calories from fat. The closer these two numbers are to each other, the more fat the food contains.

Check the ingredients for the words "hydrogenated" or "partially hydrogenated." They mean trans fat.

Percent Daily Value

The FDA has established recommended daily maximum quantities of cholesterol, salt, and fat based on a standard adult diet of 2,000 calories. The Percent Daily Value number indicates the percentage of that daily amount a single serving contains. Look for foods with 5% Daily Value or less of saturated fat per serving.

Cholesterol

This number details the amount of cholesterol in a serving. Choose foods with the lowest numbers for cholesterol. You should eat less than 200 to 300 milligrams of cholesterol a day. High intakes of dietary cholesterol raise levels of LDL cholesterol in the blood.

Claims on product packages can be confusing. By law:

- "Fat free" means less than 0.5 g fat per serving.
- "No trans fats" means less than 0.5 g trans fat per serving.
- "Low saturated fat" means 1 g saturated fat or less per serving.
- "Low fat" means a total of 3 g or less fat per serving.
- "Reduced fat" means at least 25 percent less fat than the regular version. (This may still be a lot, so check the label!)

Here's the Skinny on Fats

All fats present you with the same number of calories (nine calories per gram), but some are much better for you than others.

Saturated fats are bad for your heart because consuming them raises blood levels of LDL ("bad") cholesterol, which contributes to heart disease by clogging arteries. Common sources of saturated fats are fatty meats, whole milk and cheese, butter, lard, and palm and coconut oils.

Trans fats are a type of fat formed when liquid oils undergo a process called hydrogenation that turns them into solid fats, such as shortening and hard margarine. These hydrogenated or trans fats increase the shelf life and flavor stability of foods that contain them. In your body, however, trans fats may be even more potent than saturated fats at raising levels of LDL cholesterol. In addition, trans fats lower levels of HDL ("good" cholesterol) in the blood, making them doubly harmful when it comes to increasing heart-disease risk.

Trans fats are found in some of the same foods that contain saturated fat, such as vegetable shortenings, solid margarines, crackers, cookies, snack foods, fast-food French fries, other fried foods, and baked goods. They also show up in any processed foods that contain partially hydrogenated vegetable oils.

Saturated fat and total fats have long been included on food labels. Since January 1, 2006, the U.S. Food and Drug Administration (FDA) has required that the amount of trans fats be listed as well.

Separate listings for monounsaturated and polyunsaturated fats are not required on food labels, but some labels may list them voluntarily. Monounsaturated fats are plentiful in avocados, peanuts, and other types of nuts, as well as in olive oil and canola oil. Polyunsaturated fat comes chiefly from vegetable sources; it is the main fat in soybean oil, corn oil, and sunflower oil. (An important polyunsaturated fat known as omega-3 is found mainly in fish.)

In contrast to saturated and trans fats, monounsaturated and polyunsaturated fats don't increase levels of LDL cholesterol. When consumed in moderation, in fact, mono- and polyunsaturated fats may offer important health benefits.

Research indicates that certain forms of unsaturated fat have a beneficial effect on cholesterol levels. And some studies indicate that eating fatty fish such as salmon and mackerel—both of which are rich in polyunsaturated omega-3s—can protect against heart disease and other health problems such as arthritis. As for monounsaturated fats, olive oil—which consists mainly of monounsaturated fat—is a key part of the "Mediterranean Diet," widely recognized as a heart-healthy diet.

Opt for unsaturated fat

Whenever possible, choose foods containing unsaturated fats (those with monounsaturated or polyunsaturated fats) rather than foods with saturated or trans fats. As noted above, mono- and polyunsaturated fats don't raise LDL ("bad") cholesterol the way saturated and trans fats do, and they offer other health benefits as well.

Given the choice, you should probably go with monounsaturated fats as the healthiest type to eat. But the polyunsaturated fats offered by corn oil and other oils are good choices too—certainly far healthier than saturated or trans fats.

At least two-thirds of your total fat should be *un*saturated fat, either monounsaturated or polyunsaturated. But even these "good" fats should be eaten in moderation: At nine calories per gram, they can add a lot of calories to your diet.

Do your best to limit or eliminate saturated and trans fats in the blood. No more than 7 to 10 percent of your total calories—one-third of the total fat you eat—should be saturated fat.

Are you eating too much fat?

How do you know if you're eating too much fat? First, set your total calories for the day. (The FDA standard for an adult is 2,000 calories a day, but your number may be significantly higher or lower depending on such factors as your activity level; check with your health care provider.) Next, calculate your daily limits for total fat and saturated fat based on the recommended 30 percent and 10 percent levels, respectively, or other targets you and your doctor have determined. Then read food labels and other sources of nutritional information to help you add up the grams of total fat and saturated fat you eat. Obviously, any number over the limit means you're eating too much fat.

When Foods Lack Labels

Some foods, such as bakery items, fruits, vegetables, and meats, have no nutritional labels. You can get information on the content of these foods from various books, pamphlets, and websites. Buy a pocket-sized booklet or print a list from the Internet and take it with you when you go grocery shopping. Some lists detail the numbers for prepared meals, which you can use as a guide when you eat out.

Sodium & Fiber: Nutrients for the Heart

Nutrition labels on canned, packaged, and frozen foods also include information on two other ingredients that affect heart health: salt (or sodium) and fiber. They represent opposite extremes: Too much sodium can contribute to high blood pressure and heart disease, whereas eating plenty of fiber can improve heart health and confer many other health benefits.

Eat less sodium

If you have high blood pressure, your health care provider may tell you to eat less than 2,400 milligrams of sodium a day, which can help bring your pressure down. Here are some tips to help you decrease sodium intake:

Find the list of ingredients on the food label. (Ingredients are always listed in descending order from greatest to least amount.) Any of the following words near the top of the list warns you that the food is high in sodium:

- monosodium glutamate (MSG)
- sodium bicarbonate
- pickles or pickled
- brine
- cured
- smoked

- Buy fresh food whenever possible, or buy plain frozen food such as frozen vegetables with no butter, sauce, or other flavorings.
- Remove the salt shaker from the dining-room table and kitchen counter. Instead, season food with herbs, spices, lemon juice, or vinegar.
- Limit your use of soy sauce, steak and chili sauces, onion and garlic salt, and packaged seasoning mixes.

Before you try a salt substitute, ask your doctor if it is safe for you. Potassium chloride—a common ingredient in salt substitutes—can, in high amounts, be harmful for people taking certain drugs for high blood pressure or for heart failure.

Eat more fiber

Eating enough fiber can help lower your risk of heart disease. One kind of fiber in particular—soluble fiber—helps lower cholesterol. Both soluble and insoluble fiber may also help you control your weight. That's because high-fiber foods make you feel full longer.

Try to eat 20 to 35 grams of fiber a day. (Most people eat only about half that much.) Start by adding fiber to your diet gradually.

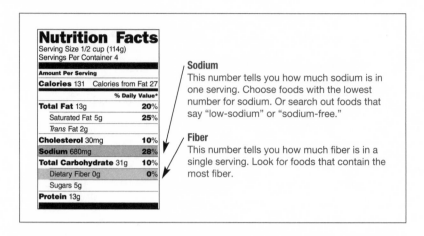

Nutrition Facts
Serving Size 1/2 cup (114g)
Servings Per Container 4

Amount Per Serving

Calories 131 Calories from Fat 27

	% Daily Value*
Total Fat 13g	**20%**
Saturated Fat 5g	**25%**
Trans Fat 2g	
Cholesterol 30mg	**10%**
Sodium 680mg	**28%**
Total Carbohydrate 31g	**10%**
Dietary Fiber 0g	**0%**
Sugars 5g	
Protein 13g	

Sodium
This number tells you how much sodium is in one serving. Choose foods with the lowest number for sodium. Or search out foods that say "low-sodium" or "sodium-free."

Fiber
This number tells you how much fiber is in a single serving. Look for foods that contain the most fiber.

This will allow your system to acclimate to the increased bulk in your intestinal tract; it can also help prevent gas.

Because fiber can absorb up to 15 times its weight in water, being on a high-fiber diet and not drinking enough fluids can lead to constipation—and, possibly, intestinal blockage. To parry this peril, drink at least eight glasses of water a day. (Check with your health care provider to guarantee this is okay for you.)

Reading food labels will help you find foods that are high in fiber. Good sources include:

- Fruits and vegetables (eat at least five servings a day)
- Whole-grain breads and cereals (make them an important part of your meals)
- Legumes such as beans and lentils (try them in soups, stews, and salads)

Patrol the Perimeter

Before you go grocery shopping, make a list. Write down the things you'll need to make healthier meals and snacks. When you get to the store, read food labels to help you choose foods that are low in fat, cholesterol, and sodium. You'll find that many of your healthiest food choices—fruits, vegetables, milk, and lean meats—are on offer in the outermost aisles of food stores. Detailed below are some ideas for healthy foods to buy.

Bread, cereal, rice, and pasta

- Whole-grain breads and rolls
- English muffins and bagels
- Whole-wheat pita bread
- Corn tortillas or rice cakes
- Oatmeal and high-fiber cold cereals
- Rice and other grains such as bulgur, couscous, corn grits, kasha, and millet
- Spaghetti, macaroni, and noodles
- Low-fat crackers, pretzels, and matzo

Limit donuts, muffins, and pastries.

Fruits and vegetables

- Fresh fruit
- Dried fruit
- Canned fruit in light syrup
- Fresh vegetables (try ready-cut to save time)
- Frozen vegetables with no added salt or sauce
- Canned vegetables with little or no sodium (check the label)

Limit coconut, olives, and avocados (olives and avocados contain beneficial monounsaturated fat but should still be consumed in moderation); vegetables in butter, cream, or cheese sauce; fruit canned in heavy syrup.

Fiber Options

All of the following foods are good sources of fiber. They are also low in fat and cholesterol. Check the foods you'd like to try:

___ Acorn squash	___ Cooked dried beans	___ Oat or wheat bran
___ Apples with skin	___ Cooked dried lentils	___ Okra
___ Artichokes	___ Cooked oatmeal	___ Oranges
___ Baked potatoes	___ Cooked split peas	___ Pears with skin
___ Barley or bulgur	___ Corn	___ Popcorn (air-popped)
___ Bran cereal	___ Dried apricots or figs	___ Prunes
___ Brown rice	___ Fresh berries	___ Pumpernickel bread
___ Brussels sprouts	___ Green peas	___ Wheat germ
___ Canned beans	___ Lima beans	___ Whole-grain breads
___ Carrots	___ Mangoes or papaya	___ Whole-wheat noodles

Meat, poultry, fish, beans, eggs, and nuts

- Lean cuts of meat (trim all visible fat)
- White-meat chicken or turkey
- Fresh fish or fish canned in water
- Tofu or tempeh (soybean cakes)
- Canned or dried beans and lentils
- Egg substitute such as EggBeaters™ or a homemade substitute

Limit bacon, liver, lunch meats, ground meat, and fish canned in oil.

Milk, yogurt, and cheese

- Nonfat or low-fat milk
- Calcium-fortified soy or rice milk
- Nonfat yogurt
- Low-fat or nonfat cottage cheese and reduced-fat cheese
- Low-fat ice cream and nonfat frozen yogurt

Limit cream, whole milk, and powdered creamers.

Fats, oils, and sweets

- Canola oil, olive oil, or liquid margarine (use sparingly)
- Spray-on cooking oils
- Light or fat-free salad dressing and mayonnaise

Limit sweets and foods made with butter or coconut, or those made with palm or hydrogenated oils.

To Buy and Try

Check the low-fat items you could add to your shopping list:

___ Corn flakes	___ Prewashed carrots	___ Chicken breasts
___ Brown rice	___ Frozen spinach	___ Olive oil cooking
___ Fresh apples	___ Tuna canned in water	spray

Which other healthful ingredients would you like to try? Write them here: _____

_____

_____

Healthful Cooking

Cooking for maximum heart health starts with cutting back on the fat and salt you add to foods. This may mean learning some new cooking methods. What it does *not* mean, however, is losing flavor or spending extra time in the kitchen. Many quick and easy cooking methods use no (or very little) fat and salt. A cookbook with low-fat, low-sodium recipes can help. So can the tips below.

Cook with less fat

Remove the skin from chicken and turkey, and trim all visible fat from meat before cooking.

- Broil, bake, stew, poach, or microwave fish, chicken, turkey, and meat.
- Brown meat under the broiler.
- Roast on a rack so the fat drips away.
- Rather than frying food in fat, simmer it in low-sodium broth or wine.
- Use nonstick pans or a nonstick cooking spray.
- Steam or microwave vegetables without adding fat or salt.
- Chill soups and stews, then skim off any fat before reheating and serving.

Add flavor without adding fat or salt

- Try herb blends, lemon juice, pepper, or flavored vinegar on vegetables.
- Add chopped onions, garlic, and hot peppers to flavor beans and rice.

- Sprinkle herbs on fish, chicken, turkey, and meat, and in soups.
- Marinate fish, chicken, turkey, and meat for added flavor. Try marinades using ginger, lemon juice, low-sodium salsa, or wine.
- Spoon natural cooking juices over meat in place of gravy or cream sauce.

Lighten up!

Replace whole milk or cream in soups and sauces with low-fat milk, evaporated skimmed milk, or nonfat dry milk.

- Replace milk or cream in puddings and other desserts with low-fat milk or fat-free condensed milk.
- Replace half the fat called for in baked goods with applesauce.
- Use low-fat or nonfat sour cream or cottage cheese to make dips and toppings.
- Use nonfat yogurt or low-fat buttermilk in salad dressings.
- Use two egg whites or ¼ cup egg substitute (such as banana or tofu) in place of one whole egg.
- Use fat-free or reduced-fat cheese in place of high-fat cheese.

Healthful Eating Out

You don't have to give up eating out to cut down on fat, cholesterol, and salt. You simply need to pause and consider what you order. Many menus highlight low-fat and low-sodium dishes. If you can't find what you want, ask. Explain to the server that you are looking for choices lower in fat, cholesterol, and salt. Or ask to see printed nutrition information. Here are some tips for ordering healthful meals.

Make your needs known

- Ask that foods be prepared in little or no fat, and with no added salt.
- Ask that sauces be left off or served on the side. Choose sauces with a tomato base rather than a cream or cheese base. Then eat only a little.
- Ask for a baked or boiled potato served plain, or steamed rice without butter.

- Ask that vegetables be steamed and served with no butter or sauce, or accompanied by lemon juice or vinegar for added flavor.

Manipulate the menu even more

- Ask about the sodium content of soup. Minestrone and vegetable soups (rather than cream-based soups) are usually the best choices.
- Order salad dressing on the side. Then use only a small amount by dipping your fork in the dressing rather than pouring the dressing over the salad.
- Look for fish, chicken, turkey, or meat that is broiled, roasted, poached, or steamed.

Try ordering one or two healthy appetizers or a low-sodium soup and a salad instead of a main dish. Or eat only half of the main dish and take the rest home.

SALAD BARS AND BUFFETS

Some healthier choices include:

- Lettuce, plain fresh vegetables, beans, fruit, and flavored gelatin
- Low-fat or fat-free salad dressing, or vinegar and a little oil
- Whole-wheat bread or bread sticks
- Roast chicken or turkey breast
- Steamed vegetables without butter or sauce
- Pasta or bean salads made with oil-and-vinegar dressing

FAST FOODS

Try these healthier orders:

- Broiled, roasted, or grilled chicken sandwich without mayonnaise, dressing, or sauce
- Chicken or whole-bean burrito or soft taco without cheese, sour cream, or guacamole
- Garden salad with light or fat-free dressing
- Baked potato with chives
- Mashed potatoes without gravy

ITALIAN

Smarter choices include:

- Minestrone soup
- Pasta with tomato sauce or sautéed vegetables (pasta primavera)
- Fish stew (cioppino)
- Chicken cacciatore
- Ravioli or tortellini in tomato sauce
- Risotto (rice) with vegetables
- Pizza with vegetable toppings and little or no cheese

MEXICAN

Make these healthier choices:

- Chicken tostada or enchilada with whole beans and no cheese, guacamole, or sour cream
- Chicken tamale
- Burrito with black beans and chicken
- Whole beans and rice
- Steamed tortillas without butter or salt
- Rice with chicken (*arroz con pollo*)
- Chicken or fish fajita

ASIAN

Look for these healthier dishes:

- Steamed, not fried, potstickers or dumplings
- Fish, chicken, or tofu stir-fried with vegetables
- Sushi or sashimi
- Steamed rice or boiled noodle dishes
- Steamed vegetable dishes
- Thai seafood stew
- Stir-fried chicken or fish with vegetables and no soy sauce

If You Smoke, Stop!

Quitting smoking is the single best thing you can do to help your heart. Why?

Because smoking is the single worst thing you can do to your arteries and to your heart.

Though legal, nicotine is every bit as addictive as heroin or cocaine. Quitting won't be easy. Even so, more than one million smokers manage to kick the habit every year— and so can you! (Indeed, grinding out butts became something of a groundswell in 2006, when smoking rates in the United States hit a 50-year low.) Once you resolve to get the monkey off your back, you may be surprised at what a wide range of sources stand ready to help you achieve that goal. But first you have to make the decision to quit for good.

Five years after kicking the habit, an ex-smoker's risk of a heart attack is no greater than that of someone who never smoked.

How Smoking Invites Heart Disease

Most people associate smoking with lung disease. But smoking is probably even more destructive as a cause of heart disease. Smoking hurts the heart—and its coronary arteries—in many basic ways:

- Toxic chemicals in smoke damage the lining of arteries, including the blood vessels that nourish the heart. This encourages artery-narrowing plaque to build up in these arteries.
- The nicotine and carbon monoxide in cigarette smoke reduce oxygen in the blood.

- Smoking stimulates the formation of blood clots that can trigger heart attacks as well as strokes.
- Smoking constricts coronary arteries, which reduces blood flow to the heart muscle.
- Smoking can increase blood pressure and make the heart beat too fast.
- Smoking blunts the protective effect of HDL cholesterol, the "good" cholesterol that helps remove the "bad" LDL cholesterol from artery walls. So smoking may be a particular problem for premenopausal women, who rely on their high HDL levels to protect them from heart disease.
- For people with heart disease, smoking can disturb the heart rhythm and lead to sudden cardiac arrest, in which the heart stops beating. Smoking is the single biggest risk factor for sudden cardiac arrest, which causes death within minutes.

Women who smoke and use oral contraceptives have a much greater risk of heart disease than women who do either activity alone.

Smoking is also the biggest risk factor for peripheral vascular disease, the narrowing of arteries that carry blood to the leg and arm muscles. In fact, peripheral vascular disease—which can lead to gangrene and leg amputation—occurs almost exclusively in smokers.

And by smoking, you put your family and friends at risk of heart disease from secondhand smoke.

The Benefits of Quitting

Now for the good news: If you quit smoking now, you can halt—and in some cases even reverse—the damaging effects of smoking detailed above. In addition, you can greatly lower the chance of suffering a first or repeat heart attack or stroke. You are definitely more likely to live a longer and healthier life if you stop smoking.

Rating Your Risk

Your risk of developing heart disease is related to the number of cigarettes you smoke and how long you've smoked. Just four cigarettes a day increases your risk of heart attack by 50 percent. One pack a day doubles your risk. And if you smoke two or more packs a day, your risk of developing heart disease is three times as high as a person who has never smoked.

Quitting for (Your) Good

If you're like most smokers, you have probably tried to quit smoking more than once. That's okay. Most people have to try several times before they quit for good. If you've tried to quit and failed, you now know what didn't work before—and that's a big advantage: You need not fall into the same traps again. This can be the time you finally break your addiction once and for all. There is no denying that quitting can be tough, but plenty of evidence from the legion of former smokers says it is not impossible.

Teetotal tips

There's no single correct way to stop smoking. What works for one person may not work for someone else—or anyone else, for that matter. But certain approaches have proved successful for most people. Some of these tips may help you:

- Quitting "cold turkey" instead of cutting back gradually seems to be the best method for most people.
- Pick a date within the next month to quit smoking entirely. Mark the date on a calendar. When the day comes, stick to it.
- Clean cigarettes out of pockets, kitchen drawers, and any other places you may have stashed them. Throw them away, along with ashtrays and lighters.
- Make a list of all the reasons you're quitting. Carry this with you. Read it when you're tempted to smoke.
- Identify triggers that can cause a relapse—these may involve certain people, places, foods, beverages, or activities.
- Ask a friend or family member who smokes to quit with you. You can support each other.
- Join a support group or a smoking-cessation class.
- Ask a close friend if you can call and talk whenever the urge to smoke is strong. Make sure that person is willing to take your call at any time of the day or night.
- See the Appendix for additional resources.

Don't flip if you slip

A lapse doesn't mean you've lost. Look at it as a chance to learn. If you find the reason for your slip, you can make a plan to deal with it. Ask yourself some questions, such as:

- What was I doing when I smoked?
- Was I with a smoker?
- Was I lonely?
- What did I learn about being tempted?
- How can I avoid backsliding this way again?

If you do slip up, get right back on course. Anytime you revert to smoking, seize control of the situation by stubbing the cigarette out. Capitalize on the moment to keep yourself from falling back into your old smoking pattern. If you tried to quit before and didn't succeed, don't doubt yourself this time. Use what you've learned to help keep yourself in your new nonsmoking pattern.

Track your triggers

If you are still smoking, do you find that certain emotions, such as anger, trigger your urge to smoke? Certain people or places? Certain drinks such as coffee or alcohol? Knowing the situations that make you want to smoke can arm you against slipups after you quit. To track your triggers, fold a piece of paper and slip it inside your pack of cigarettes. For one day, record the time of day you smoked each cigarette, anything noteworthy about the circumstance, and your feelings just before you lit up. Do any patterns emerge?

Smokers 60 or older can add 5 to 7 years to their lives by quitting.

Once you've identified triggers that cause you to light up, try to think of actions that might help divert you from smoking. If you reach for a cigarette as soon as you wake up, for example, substitute another first-thing-in-the-morning action such as brushing your teeth or making the bed. If drinking coffee triggers the smoking urge, try drinking tea or juice instead. If cigarettes are your stress reliever at work, practice deep breathing exercises during your break.

Coping with urges

It's normal to keep feeling the urge to smoke once you quit. The goal is to find ways to beat your triggers. Substituting alternative actions for smoking when triggering events occur is one good approach. Here are some other useful tactics for dealing with—or outright avoiding—your triggers.

- Realize that your urge to smoke will pass within about five minutes. During that time, keep busy by taking a walk, reading a book or magazine, talking to a friend, or drinking something nonalcoholic. (For many people, drinking an alcoholic beverage triggers the desire to smoke.)
- Keep your hands busy by doodling or twisting a paper clip, knitting—anything so that you won't miss holding a cigarette.
- A trick that works for some people: Hold and even take drags on an unlit cigarette when the smoking urge hits. That provides the "oral fixation" that smokers crave, plus the familiar manual manipulation of the cigarette—everything except actually inhaling the nicotine and smoke.
- Keep your mouth busy with a straw or toothpick or by munching carrot sticks or chewing gum.
- Sit in nonsmoking areas of restaurants so you don't see or smell smoke.
- Ask a friend if you can call and talk whenever the craving for a cigarette strikes.
- Find and join a support group of fellow quitters.
- Get phone counseling from a "quit" help line.

Try these relaxation techniques

People often smoke in an effort to deal with unpleasant emotions. You might find that you smoke when you feel stressed, for example, or when you feel impatient, frustrated, or angry. Learning relaxation skills can help. Instead of reaching for a cigarette, try deep breathing:

- Take a deep breath.
- Feel your lungs, chest, and diaphragm stretch and expand.

- Exhale slowly.
- Repeat several times until you feel calmer.

Deep breathing is a simple tool that you can use anytime to help banish the urge to smoke. You may also want to try yoga, stretching, or other relaxation activities.

Products that can help

Smoking-cessation products lessen your urge to light up. Most replace nicotine for a while. All help you ease off your addiction. Combined with counseling, any of the products listed on page 131 can double your chances of long-term success. Some are available over the counter; for others you will need a prescription. Think about which of these you'd like to try, then discuss your choices with your doctor. For best results, make sure you take any nicotine-replacement product for the recommended time period.

If you choose an over-the-counter product, talk to your pharmacist and read the label carefully. As soon as you can, tell your doctor which over-the-counter product you're using.

Be Smart for Your Heart

Now is the time to take steps to reduce your risk of heart disease and heart attack. It may take a while to change your habits, but the rewards will be worth the effort. You'll still enjoy eating—and you'll feel better, too. Here's what you need to do:

- Limit the amount of fat, cholesterol, and salt you eat.
- Read food labels and use the food pyramid (see pages 110–114) to help you choose foods that are low in fat and high in fiber.
- Eat the right number of calories to stay at a healthy weight.
- Get some physical activity almost every day.

The Very Low Fat Cardiac Diet: Worth the Effort?

Guidelines from the American Heart Association and the National Cholesterol Education Program have set a standard of 30 percent or less of total calories from fat. But people with life-threatening heart

	How It Works	Length of Treatment	Some Possible Side Effects
Over-the-Counter			
Nicotine Patch	•Gives you nicotine through the skin at a constant rate •Ask your doctor about combining the patch with nicotine gum or nasal spray	Take decreasing dosages over about two months	•Skin rash, itching •Insomnia •Nausea •Dry mouth
Nicotine Gum	•Gives you nicotine through the mouth	Take decreasing dosages over two to three months	•Sore mouth or jaw •Indigestion •Dizziness, nausea
Nicotine Lozenge	•Gives you nicotine through the mouth	Take decreasing dosages over about three months	•Sore mouth •Belching •Dizziness, nausea, weakness
Prescription Only			
Nicotine Nasal Spray	•Gives you nicotine through the nose •Works more quickly than other nicotine products	Use for three to six months	•Irritated nose, eyes, throat •Coughing, sneezing
Inhaler	•Nicotine is breathed in through the mouth (similar to a cigarette)	Use for up to six months	•Mouth and throat irritation •Coughing
Bupropion SR	•Reduces smoking urges and withdrawal symptoms •Does not contain nicotine	Start two weeks before you quit, then take for two to six months	•Insomnia •Dry mouth •Shakiness •Skin rash

NOTE: Each product listed conflicts with certain other medications or certain medical conditions. If you have questions, ask your pharmacist or doctor. Don't smoke while using a nicotine product. Doing so can give you a dangerous overdose of nicotine.

conditions (those who have already experienced a heart attack, for example) may want to consider lowering their fat intake even more—to less than 15 percent of calories from fat.

This very low fat diet is essentially a diet that excludes animal products. Although adopting such a diet may seem difficult, surveys indicate that heart patients placed on low-fat vegetarian diets find them highly acceptable. Even more important, research shows that such diets can help to halt and even reverse the artery clogging that occurs in heart disease.

Weight: Your Loss Is Your Gain

Calories are the fuel your body burns for energy. You get these calories from food. When you eat more calories than you need for your activity level, however, your body stores the extra calories as fat and you gain weight.

Too much extra weight can raise your blood pressure and cholesterol, and it increases your risk of developing diabetes. So losing pounds if you're overweight is vitally important. But how to do it? Behind all the gimmicks and fad diets out there is one unchanging truth: The only way to lose weight is to burn, or use up, more calories than you take in. And the best way to do that is to combine regular exercise with a healthy diet.

Should you lose weight?

If you're overweight, your risk of developing high blood pressure is two to six times what if would be if you were at a normal weight.

The standard method of telling whether you're overweight is to calculate your body mass index (BMI), a number determined by taking your height and weight into account. If you want to do the math, divide your weight in pounds by the square of your height in inches, then multiply this result by 703. Or simply consult the BMI chart on page 53.

Choose what to lose

The amount of weight you should lose depends, of course, on how much you now weigh and how much you should weigh. Work with your health care provider to set safe, realistic weight-loss goals. Research shows that overweight people can generally improve their health by losing 5 to 15 percent of their body weight in a slow and steady fashion.

A flab-shedding stratagem

To lose weight safely and keep it off, you need to eat fewer calories *and* become more active. Lasting weight loss, though difficult, is feasible. But you must have a plan. Try this one:

- Work with your health care provider to set a weight goal and schedule. It's best to lose weight slowly and steadily.
- Reduce your daily intake of calories. Keep a list of what you eat and read food labels and other sources of nutritional information to calculate how many calories you consume daily (see page 136).

- Become more active, which will cause you to burn more calories. By combining calorie reduction with increased activity, you force your body to start burning the extra calories that are stored as fat.
- Track your progress. Weigh yourself once a week. (Daily weigh-ins aren't necessary; indeed, they can be counterproductive, since day-to-day fluctuations in weight can make people anxious.) Keep a record of the results in a log or diary so you can gauge how well your weight-loss plan is working. Adjust your activity level and caloric intake as necessary to reach your goals on schedule.

Reading food labels

The first step toward weight loss is to learn how many calories you're consuming, and the best way to see what's really in the food you eat is to read labels. Although the "Nutrition Facts" food label was discussed earlier in this chapter in the context of fats, it bears reexamination here—this time focusing on the nutrition data that are most important for people who want to reduce their caloric intake and lose weight. (Note: All food labels include "Percent Daily Value" figures for nutritional elements, but they are based on a 2,000-calorie diet—and may therefore not be helpful if your diet calls for more or fewer calories. The other numbers on the label, however, provide all the information you need.)

In the U.S., 65 percent of adults are now considered overweight. In 1995, by contrast, only 56 percent of U.S. adults were overweight.

SERVING SIZE

This tells you how much is in a single serving whether it's ounces or grams or numbers of units. All the values on the label are based on this amount. Keep two key things in mind: First, be aware that one serving is often less than what a person would normally consume. If, for example, you eat four cookies and a single serving consists of only two, you will need to double all the values on the label. Second, be sure to check the number of servings a package or container holds. Many products that you might reasonably expect to consume

Nutrition Facts

Serving size 2 cookies
Servings per container 6

Amount Per Serving

Calories 140   **Calories from Fat** 70

	% Daily Value*
Total Fat 7g	11%
Saturated Fat 2.5g	13%
Trans Fat 3g	
Cholesterol 10mg	3%
Sodium 105mg	4%
Total Carbohydrates 16g	5%
Dietary Fiber 1g	4%
Sugars 5g	
Protein 2g	

Vitamin A 0%	●	**Vitamin C** 0%	
Calcium 0%	●	**Iron**	2%

*Percent Daily Values are based on a 2,000 calorie diet.

INGREDIENTS: UNBLEACHED ENRICHED WHEAT FLOUR [FLOUR, NIACIN, REDUCED IRON, THIAMINE MONONITRATE (VITAMIN B1), RIBOFLAVIN (VITAMIN B2), FOLIC ACID], PARTIALLY HYDROGENATED VEGETABLE SHORTENING (SOYBEAN AND COTTONSEED OILS), SUGAR, BUTTER, CORNSTARCH, INVERT SUGAR, CONTAINS 2 PERCENT OR LESS OF: NONFAT MILK, EGG WHITES, SALT, AND BAKING SODA.

in a single sitting contain more than one serving; a regular 6-ounce can of tuna, for example, has 2.5 servings. Again, you'll have to multiply all the other values on the label to find your totals.

CALORIES

This shows the total number of calories in a single serving. If you compare a few labels, you may see that many foods called "low sugar," "low carb" (for "low carbohydrate"), and even "low fat" are actually high in calories. As you monitor your other dietary needs, don't forget that your calorie total is the crucial number determining whether or not you'll lose weight. It's also important not to go too far. For healthy weight loss, women should eat no fewer than 1,200 calories a day; men should eat no fewer than 1,500 calories a day. (Eating less than this deprives your body of its minimum energy requirements.)

CALORIES FROM FAT

This tells you how many calories per serving come from fat. The closer this number is to the total calories, the more fat the food contains. Reducing overall calories is your goal, but fat calories also need to be held in check for a variety of health reasons—among them the fact that your body is more likely to store these calories as fat.

TOTAL FAT

You'll see here the weight in grams of the fat in a single serving. Foods high in fat are also high in calories because 1 g of fat has 9 calories, whereas 1 g of protein or carbohydrate has only 4 calories. Keep your total fat below 3 g per 100 calories; this ensures less than 30 percent of your calories come from fat. Eating too much of certain fats also puts you at higher risk of heart disease. Look for:

- Saturated fat: 1 g or less per 100 calories, to keep your daily amount below 10 percent of your total calories.
- Trans fat: As little as possible. Although the FDA has not set a daily value percentage for trans fat, any amount is detrimental because trans fats raise LDL ("bad") cholesterol.
- Hydrogenated oils: Look for these in the ingredients list; you may also see the term "partially hydrogenated." These oils, which have had hydrogen added to them, are the source of trans fats and should be avoided whenever possible.
- Dietary fiber: High-fiber foods are digested more slowly than lower-fiber foods, meaning you feel full longer and tend to want to eat less. Try to get an average of 25 to 35 g of fiber per day.

Assembling a healthy meal

To lose weight, you can eat just about anything you want—so long as you don't eat too much of it. But beware any diet that focuses on a single type of food; such regimens are notoriously difficult to observe for more than a few weeks, and many of them are downright unhealthy. Over time, you will be healthier eating a variety of foods.

Losing excess weight reduces your risk of heart disease by lowering LDL ("bad" cholesterol) and raising HDL ("good" cholesterol).

Try to plan meals around grains, vegetables, and fruits. Limit meat and other fatty foods. You can use the plate model shown below as a guide. When you put food on your plate, cover:

- At least half of the plate with vegetables and fruits.
- A quarter with whole grains or other unrefined carbohydrates, such as brown rice.
- No more than a quarter with fish, meat, poultry, or other sources of protein.

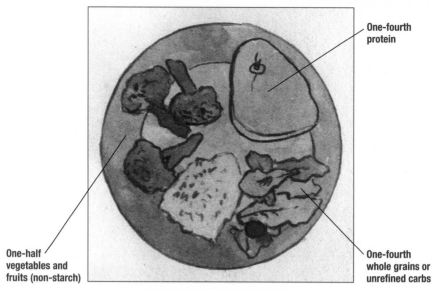

One-fourth protein

One-half vegetables and fruits (non-starch)

One-fourth whole grains or unrefined carbs

> The Filling Fractions of a Model Plate

Draw up a food diary

Try keeping a food diary for three or more days (including at least one weekend day); a week is ideal. Write down all the food and drink you consume. Include how much of the food or drink you have and how many calories it contains. Also write down the time of day, where you are, and what you're doing—besides eating, that is!

One large study found that losing just 10 pounds lowers systolic blood pressure (the top number) by nearly 4 mm Hg and diastolic pressure (the bottom number) by nearly 3 mm Hg.

Tracking not only what you eat but also when, where, and why may help you spot patterns in your eating habits. You may find that when you're watching TV or reading a book, for example, you snack despite not being hungry. Or perhaps you always pick up a candy bar when you go in to pay for gas. You may discover ways to cut calories just by changing certain facets of your routine. Keep a bottle of water handy to sip from as you watch TV or read, for instance, or pay at the pump instead of subjecting yourself to that tempting display of munchies inside the station.

Forgo fads

Most of us have been tempted to try a fad diet at one time or another. Here's the glitch: Fad diets aim at quick weight loss and thus focus on changing how you eat for only a short period of time. They do not help you keep the weight off. If you don't continue to balance the calories you eat with the calories you burn, you'll regain the weight once the diet is over.

To reach and maintain a healthy weight, you must permanently change your eating and lifestyle habits. Rather than gambling with fads, work with your health care provider or a dietitian to develop a safe, sustainable plan for weight loss. Remember, you're in this for the long haul.

> Body shape matters when it comes to being overweight. People shaped like apples (carrying excess weight in the abdomen) face a greater risk of developing diabetes and heart disease than those shaped like pears (fat deposits in the hips, thighs, and buttocks).

Less Stress Is Best

You most likely know that stress plays an important role in heart disease. Chronic stress can increase your heart rate, blood pressure, and blood-sugar levels; it may also cause damage to the walls of your arteries. What you may not know is that you can manage stress so it doesn't take a toll on your heart.

What Is Stress?

Stress is the way your body and mind react to demands and changing circumstances. When you're under stress, your heart rate and blood pressure go up—a genetically programmed reaction known as the fight-or-flight response that prepares the body for sudden action. Too much stress over an extended period of time can cause physical damage to your heart and circulatory system; it can also affect your behavior in ways detrimental to your health.

Choosing Your Response

You can control the effects of stress by changing the way you respond to the factors in your life that cause stress. The key is to know what these so-called stressors are. Try keeping a stress diary for a few weeks. Make a note of anything that causes you to feel tense or "stressed out," and also note how you react to each identified stressor. You may find that you fall into unhealthy habits when-

Stress affects each person differently. Below are some signs of stress. Check off the ways in which you respond to stress:

___Headaches | ___Impatience | ___Drinking more or
___Upset stomach/ | ___Depression | using drugs
   heartburn | ___Low self-esteem | ___Smoking more
___Sweating | ___Forgetfulness | ___Becoming accident-
___Frequent colds | ___Trouble | prone
___Skin problems | concentrating |
___Sexual problems | ___Overeating |
___Anger | ___Undereating |

ever you feel stressed; you may skip exercise, eat poorly, or smoke, further increasing your risk for heart disease. These are your soon-to-be-former responses to the stressors in your life. Now you're ready to choose new responses that combat stress without threatening your health.

No matter what the stressor is, you can take action to reduce or even eliminate it.

- Avoid it: If you find that watching the local news on TV makes you feel stressed, change the channel. Also, avoid confrontation when you can.
- Alter it: Join a carpool if you don't like driving. Ask someone to do something in a new way if the old way raises your stress level.
- Adapt to it: Sometimes you can neither avoid nor change a stressor. But you can control it by adapting to it. Try to think about it in a new way. And try to accept the things you can't alter.

Slow thyself

When faced with a stressor, ask yourself these questions:

- How much will this matter in a year?
- Is this worth getting upset about?
- What can I gain from this experience? (Perhaps being stuck in traffic gives you time to listen to music or a book on tape.)
- What are the good things in my life? (Try to switch your focus to something pleasant.)

Preventing & Relieving Stress

The techniques described on the next few pages can help prevent stress and its harmful effects. Focusing your priorities can also save you time—another way to reduce stress in your life. And when you do feel stress, deep breathing and relaxation exercises can help calm you down.

Relaxation: a learned art

Try to spend a few minutes each day relaxing. Relaxation techniques such as yoga and meditation can slow your heart rate, bring your blood pressure down, and relax your muscles. Deep breathing is a common technique you can use anywhere.

Set priorities

Try not to worry about tasks you can't attend to right away. Decide what's most important and accomplish those items first. Look for ways to do things with less effort. Ask yourself:

- Do I really need to do this today? (It's okay to say "No," but if the answer is "Yes," take care of that chore first.)
- What do I need help with? Is there someone else who can do it?
- Can I cancel or change this appointment or social event to another time?

Exercise daily

Just about any form of exercise can help reduce stress. Talk with your health care provider about the kinds of exercise that are safe for you. Exercising with a friend may relieve your stress even more.

More stress lesseners

There are many steps you can take to shrink your overall level of stress. Try some of the following:

- Get some exercise every day.
- Make time to relax on a daily basis.
- Try to reduce the noise levels to which you're exposed.
- Spend some time alone every day.

- Keep consistent sleeping hours.
- Budget both your money and your time.
- Learn when to say "No."
- Write appointments on a calendar.
- Take a lot of mini-breaks.
- Ask for help when you need it.
- Focus on the good things in your life.
- Find hobbies you enjoy.
- Do something nice for a friend.
- Laugh whenever you can.

If you're overwhelmed or depressed and nothing seems to help, find a friend, psychiatrist, psychologist, member of the clergy, or counselor to talk to.

Combining Lifestyle Measures to Control Hypertension & Cholesterol

Smoking cessation, a healthy diet, weight loss, exercise, stress reduction—each one of these key lifestyle changes has been proven to mitigate your risk factors and help stave off heart disease. So it follows that combining several lifestyle changes can dramatically blunt two of the most important heart-disease risk factors: hypertension, or high blood pressure, and high blood-cholesterol levels.

Lifestyle Changes to Combat Hypertension

As Chapter 3 made clear, hypertension can wreak havoc with the circulatory system—and with the heart in particular. High blood pressure greatly increases your chances of having a heart attack or stroke, of suffering heart or kidney failure, and of developing Alzheimer's disease. Millions of people with hypertension require drugs to lower their blood pressure to an acceptable level and keep it there. For countless others, though, high blood pressure is reversible without medication.

More and more studies indicate that lifestyle changes can help lower blood pressure—and that such shifts can even keep hypertension from developing in the first place. If you do need drugs to control hypertension, adopting these lifestyle changes may let you lower your dose, reducing the side effects these drugs sometimes cause.

As it turns out, hypertension responds positively to all of the lifestyle changes described in this chapter, notably these:

- **Exercise briskly**. . . because exercise demonstrably lowers blood pressure. A recent study analyzing 54 exercise trials concluded that moderately aerobic workouts—brisk walking, for example—can lower blood pressure in people with hypertension by an average of 5 mm Hg systolic and 4 mm Hg diastolic.
- **Eat healthier**. . . because doing so helps reduce blood pressure and plaque buildup. Focus on two areas: Eat a diet high in fruits and vegetables and low in fat, and limit the salt in your diet.
- **Quit smoking**. . . because smoking increases blood pressure and damages blood vessels.
- **Lose weight**. . . because losing excess weight helps lower blood pressure. Weight loss can also make you feel better.
- **Reduce stress**. . . because stress can raise your blood pressure. Studies have shown that stress reduction can help people with hypertension lower their blood pressure.

Dietary Approach to Stop Hypertension (DASH)

Population studies over many years have indicated that people who eat lots of fruits and vegetables and little fat have lower blood pressure. Eager to gauge the scientific basis of this dietary approach, researchers at five leading U.S. hospitals launched a clinical trial known as DASH (Dietary Approach to Stop Hypertension).

The results of DASH—confirmed in a follow-up study—demonstrated that a diet high in fruits, vegetables, whole grains, and low-fat dairy products could indeed lower blood-pressure levels considerably. Overall, the two studies indicate that people with hypertension who adopt the DASH diet can lower their blood pressure by about 8

> More than 1 in 4 American adults have high blood pressure.

mm Hg systolic and 4 mm Hg diastolic—results that rival the effects of some antihypertensive drugs.

People with hypertension should avoid
very intense aerobic
exercise; it can force
blood pressure
to dangerously
high levels.
The table on the opposite page summarizes the DASH Eating Plan. For most people, adopting the DASH diet means substantially altering the way they eat. But if you have high blood pressure, it may be worth giving DASH a try: The diet not only reduces blood pressure but also helps lower cholesterol levels and offers numerous other health benefits, including a possible reduction in cancer risk. To learn more about the DASH Eating Plan, visit www.nhlbi.nih.gov /health/public/heart/hbp/dash.

Less salt = lower pressure

The dangers of consuming too much sodium are well known. Even if you're on medication to lower your blood pressure, cutting back on salt will improve your health and make you feel better. Adjusting to the change takes time. But you really can retrain your taste buds.

THE CASE OF THE STEALTHY SODIUM

To cut back on sodium—a mineral common in many foods—you first must know where to find it. Your taste buds tell you that certain foods are salty. But sodium also "hides" in foods that do not taste obviously salty. Here are a few food items in which you sodium lurks:

- Canned, processed, and frozen foods, such as soups, lunch meats, frozen pizza, and vegetable juice
- Mixes, such as gravy mix and instant mashed potatoes
- Pickled, cured, and smoked foods, such as relishes, bacon, and sausage
- Salty snacks, such as chips and salted popcorn
- Most fast foods, such as cheeseburgers, burritos, fries, and even chicken sandwiches
- Items that fizz in water, such as some over-the-counter medicines

The DASH Eating Plan				
Food Group	Servings	Serving Sizes	What a Serving Looks Like	Examples
Vegetables	4–5 per day	1 cup raw leafy vegetable ½ cup cooked vegetable 6 oz. vegetable juice	1 cup A fist	Tomatoes, potatoes, carrots, green peas, squash, broccoli, turnip greens, collards, kale, spinach, artichokes, green beans, lima beans, sweet potatoes
Fruits	4–5 per day	6 oz. fruit juice 1 medium fruit ¼ cup dried fruit ½ cup fresh, frozen, or canned fruit	1 medium fruit A fist	Apricots, bananas, cantaloupe, dates, grapes, oranges, orange juice, mangoes, melons, peaches, pineapples, prunes, raisins, strawberries, tangerines
Grains and grain products	7–8 per day	1 slice bread 1 oz. dry cereal ½ cup cooked rice, pasta, or cereal	½ cup A cupped hand	Whole-wheat bread, English muffin, pita bread, bagel, cereals, grits, oatmeal, unsalted pretzels, unsalted popcorn
Low-fat or fat-free dairy foods	2–3 per day	8 oz. milk 1 cup yogurt 1½ oz. cheese	1 cup A fist	Fat-free (skim) or low-fat (1%) milk, fat-free or low-fat cheese, and fat-free or low-fat regular or frozen yogurt
Meats, poultry, and fish	2 or fewer per day	3 oz. cooked meats, poultry, or fish	2 to 3 oz. A small palm	Select only lean meats. Trim away visible fat. Broil, roast, or boil instead of frying. Remove skin from poultry.
Nuts, seeds, and dry beans	4–5 per week	⅓ cup (or 1½ oz.) nuts 2 tablespoons (or ½ oz.) seeds ½ cup cooked dry beans or peas	½ cup A cupped hand	Unsalted almonds, filberts, mixed nuts, peanuts, walnuts, sunflower seeds, kidney beans, lentils
Fats and oils	2–3 per day	1 teaspoon soft margarine or vegetable oil 1 tablespoon low-fat mayonnaise 2 tablespoons light salad dressing	1 teaspoon The tip of the thumb	Vegetable oil (such as olive, corn, canola, or safflower), soft margarine, low-fat mayonnaise, light salad dressing
Sweets	No more than 5 per week	1 tablespoon sugar 1 tablespoon jelly ½ oz. jelly beans 8 oz. lemonade	1 tablespoon A thumb (from the knuckle)	Maple syrup, sugar, jelly, jam, fruit-flavored gelatin, jelly beans, hard candy, fruit punch, sorbet, flavored ices

TO CUT DOWN ON SALT

Reducing salt means adopting new shopping habits and cooking techniques. Read food labels when you shop; put high-sodium foods back on the shelf. At home, you can cut out even more sodium by preparing your food with alternative flavorings, such as herbs, pepper and other spices, lemon juice, and vinegar.

WHAT PACKAGING EXPOSES

Food labels tell you how much sodium you're getting before you even reach for the salt shaker. Don't ignore claims on the front of the box, such as "low sodium": They have exact meanings that you can learn to interpret with a little practice (see "Decoding sodium statements," below).

Check the serving size and the number of servings per container. This is the foundation for all the other values on the label. On the soup label opposite, for instance, one serving is only half the can. If you eat the whole can, you'll have to double all other figures on the label.

- Sodium is given in milligrams (mg), a unit of weight. Remember your daily goal when choosing foods.
- % Daily Value indicates the percentage of the standard recommended amount per day, so one serving of this soup contains 37 percent of the daily sodium allowance (2,400 mg).
- Scrutinize the ingredients for salt. Keep an eye peeled for such high-sodium items as sodium phosphate and monosodium glutamate (MSG).

Decoding sodium statements

Though claims on product packages can be confusing, they do have precise meanings. By law:

- "Sodium free" or "salt free" means less than 5 mg per serving.
- "Very low sodium" means 35 mg or less per serving.
- "Low sodium" means 140 mg or less per serving.
- "Reduced sodium" or "less sodium" means at least 25 percent less sodium than the standard version. (Check the label for exactly how much less.)

Make sure to check the serving size. This is the basis for all values on the label. In this case, one serving is half a can of soup. If you eat the whole can, you have to double the other numbers on the label, too.

Nutrition Facts

Serving size 1 cup
Servings per container 2

Amount Per Serving

Calories 90	Calories from fat 20

	% Daily Value
Total fat 2g	3%
Saturated fat 0g	
Cholesterol 10mg	3%
Sodium 890mg	37%
Total Carbohydrates 13g	4%
Dietary fiber 1g	4%
Sugars 1g	
Protein 6g	

Ingredients: Chicken broth, carrots, cooked white chicken meat (white chicken meat, water, salt, sodium phosphate, isolated soy protein, modified corn starch, corn starch), potatoes, celery, rice, monosodium glutamate.

Percent Daily Value gives the percentage of the standard recommended amount per day. One serving of this food therefore has 37% of a 2,400-mg daily sodium allowance.

Sodium is given in milligrams (mg), a unit of weight. Remember your daily goal when choosing foods.

Check the ingredients list for salt. Also watch for high-sodium ingredients such as monosodium glutamate (MSG), baking soda, and sodium phosphate.

- "Light in sodium" means 50 percent less sodium than the standard version. (Again, check the label for exactly how much less.)
- "Unsalted" or "no salt added" means no salt was added to the product during processing. It does not mean the product contains no salt. (You guessed it: Check the label.)
- "Healthy" and "natural" have no nutritional meaning. Don't be fooled into thinking these foods must be good for you just because their labels make that boast.

Desalinization starts at the store

Most people shop by habit, reaching for familiar items and paying scant attention to what they're putting in the basket. If you want to get serious about reducing salt and improving your diet, it's time to turn off the automatic pilot. Avoid impulse buys. Make a shopping list before you go to the store. The following tips can help you lower the sodium content of your food purchases.

- In the produce section: Start your shopping here, where you'll find lots of delicious low-sodium foods. Fresh fruits and vegetables contain almost no sodium.
- At the meat counter: Look for fresh fish, chicken, and meats. Avoid anything that's cured or smoked. Even frozen meats can have added sodium. If you're not sure, ask at the counter.
- In the frozen-food section: Frozen meals can be high in sodium. Look for plain frozen foods without sauces.
- In the snack-food section: These foods are the highest in sodium. Read labels carefully. Look for low-salt versions of your favorite snacks or find new alternatives.
- In the canned- and packaged-food aisles: Remember that processed foods are often high in sodium. Always check the label, keeping your daily goal in mind.

Tips for cooking without sodium

Pick at least two tips you'd like to try this week. The more you try, the faster your taste buds will adjust. Before too long, the foods you once favored will taste too salty.

- Put the salt shaker away; you'll use less salt than if you leave it conveniently within reach on the table or next to the stove.
- Don't salt cooking water or add salt while making meals. If you must use salt, add it to taste at the table.
- If you use canned vegetables, rinse them well to remove excess sodium.
- Use plain garlic and onion powder instead of the salted versions.
- Use sodium-free baking powder.
- Use fresh or dried herbs and spices rather than packaged seasoning mixes.
- Use half (or less than half) of the salt that a recipe calls for.
- Use only small amounts of ketchup, relish, chili sauce, and soy sauce, all of which contain salt. Try reduced-sodium versions.

What can you choose instead?

There are lots of foods that can give you the taste or texture you crave—without overloading you with sodium. Try making one change per day. Work up to making one change per meal. Of course, what you choose depends on your taste. Can you think of more alternatives for the foods you often eat?

Lifestyle Changes to Combat Cholesterol

The higher your blood cholesterol, the greater your risk for heart attack and stroke. That's why you need to know your cholesterol level. If it's high, you can take steps to lower it. If it's normal, learn how to keep it that way. Two important lifestyle measures—eating the right foods and getting regular exercise—can help bring high cholesterol levels down.

When it comes to controlling cholesterol through diet, your focus should be on two tactics in particular: eating less fat and cholesterol, and eating more fiber.

Lowering your blood pressure, whether with medication or through lifestyle changes, can reduce and even halt further arterial damage.

Pare back fat and cholesterol

Your body turns the saturated fat and dietary cholesterol you eat into blood cholesterol. The first step to lowering your cholesterol is cutting down on these:

- **Saturated fat:** This type of fat is found mainly in foods that come from animals. Such foods include meat, chicken skin, cheese, whole milk, and butter. Coconut oil, cocoa butter, palm kernel oil, and palm oil are also saturated fats.

- **Trans fats:** These fats are formed when unsaturated vegetable oils are "thickened" by the addition of hydrogen. This process, called hydrogenation, makes oils more solid (as in stick or tub margarine) and helps prevent spoilage. The resulting trans fats are considered even worse for arteries than saturated fats. They do double damage in that they increase LDL ("bad" cholesterol) and decrease HDL ("good" cholesterol). Ingredients you should avoid because of their high trans-fat content include vegetable shortening and partially hydrogenated vegetable oils. Since January of 2006, the FDA has required manufacturers to list the trans-fat content of their products.

• **Dietary cholesterol**: This is found only in foods that come from animals. Sources include eggs, liver, meats, and shellfish. Try to eat no more than 200 mg of dietary cholesterol per day. In general, don't eat more than four egg yolks a week; limit meat and poultry to no more than 6 ounces per day. Cholesterol-rich organ meats such as liver, brains, and kidneys should likewise be avoided.

If You Often Eat	Try Instead
Breakfast	
• Packaged breakfast pastries or frozen waffles	• Toasted raisin bread
• Salted butter	• Unsalted butter
• Flavored oatmeal, grits, or other cooked cereal	• Plain cooked cereal (homemade seasoning)
• Vegetable juice	• Fruit juice or low-sodium vegetable juice
• Frozen hash browns	• Fresh hash browns, or a low-sodium frozen brand
Lunch	
• Pickles	• Raw fresh vegetables
• Lunch meat or salami	• Plain sliced turkey, chicken, or beef
• Noodle soup with flavor packet	• Plain noodles (homemade seasoning)
• Processed cheese (American)	• Natural cheese (cheddar, Swiss, etc.)
• Salted chips or fries	• Unsalted pretzels, nuts, or chips
• Candy bar with nuts or caramel	• Plain chocolate bar
Dinner	
• Table salt (for cooking)	• Lemon, garlic, spices, low-sodium spice mixes
• Soy sauce	• Low-sodium soy sauce
• Bottled salad dressing	• Oil, vinegar, and herbs
• Rice dish mix	• Plain rice (homemade seasoning)
• Canned vegetables or beans	• Frozen, fresh, or low-sodium canned vegetables or beans
• Frozen potatoes or instant mashed potatoes	• Boiled or baked potatoes
• Ham	• Roast pork
• Smoked turkey	• Roast turkey or chicken
• Sausage	• Lean hamburger patty
• Ice cream	• Frozen yogurt or "light" ice cream

Eat more fiber

Eating plenty of fiber can help reduce blood cholesterol. Try consuming more oats, dried beans, brown rice, vegetables, and fruit. The best kind of fiber for lowering cholesterol levels is so-called soluble fiber, which is found in foods such as oat bran and fruits. Soluble fiber can significantly lower your blood cholesterol, particularly when it is incorporated in a low-fat diet.

Exercise early and often

Engaging in regular exercise has the very positive effect of raising your HDL ("good" cholesterol). It also helps you lose weight, which can lower your LDL ("bad" cholesterol). Walking, swimming, or cycling are all good ways to be active. As always, check with your doctor before starting any exercise program.

When 6
You Need
Treatment

RY AS YOU MIGHT, sometimes you can't control either the risk factors for heart disease or the disease itself solely with diet, exercise, and modifications to your lifestyle. When medical intervention becomes the only prudent course, you and your health care team will discuss a variety of options, some of which are relatively simple, requiring little more than regular treatment with medications. In other cases, the best choice involves a medical procedure or surgery.

This chapter describes the wide range of medical treatments currently available. The more you know about them, the better prepared you'll be to work with your doctor and other medical specialists—and the less intimidated you'll be by even the most complex and serious approaches.

Medications

Whether you need treatment for risk factors or a diagnosed heart problem, any medicines your doctor prescribes should be part of—not a substitute for—a complete program that centers on becoming more active and eating healthier foods. Be sure to talk to your health care team about developing just such a program.

It's important to educate yourself about the medications you will be taking. First and foremost, of course, you need to take each one as directed, so if you don't understand the instructions, ask your doctor or pharmacist. Many people find it helpful to translate the bottle's directions ("Take two pills three times a day with food," for

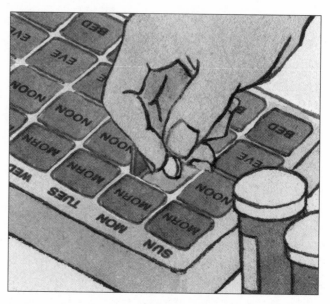

> To keep track of medications, use a pill box with day and time compartments.

example) into a schedule listing all your pills so you will know to take the right medicines at the right times (see chart on opposite page). Or, as shown above, you can use a pill box.

Over time, your doctor may change the medications you take, as well as their dosages, after a follow-up visit or routine evaluation. This is normal; just remember to update your medication schedule. Here are some more basic tips:

- You may have more than one doctor treating you. Give each of your health care providers a complete list of the medications and dosages you take. Include any herbs, supplements, and other over-the-counter (nonprescription) products. Carry a copy of this list with you in case of emergencies.
- Ask about any known interactions between the medications you're taking—including nonprescription products. Know when and how to take each medication, and follow the directions about whether you need to take it with food or on an empty stomach.
- Refill each prescription well before the time you would run out.

My Medication Chart

Fill in the chart below to keep track of all your medications. Any time your doctor adds a medication, tells you to stop one, or changes a dosage, record the change here. Share this list among your doctors (if you have more than one) and with any new health care provider you visit. Keep a copy in your wallet or purse.

Generic Name	Brand Name (if any)	Strength (dose)	Quantity per dose	How often to Take	Purpose	Notes
Sample Med	Sample Brand	25mg	1 pill	Once a day	Lower cholesterol	Bedtime. No grapefruit Rx by Dr. Carter.

List also all the vitamins, minerals, herbs, and supplements you are taking.

_____

_____

_____

_____

- Never stop taking a medication without talking to your doctor first. Stopping a medication suddenly could raise your blood pressure or heart rate, or cause other serious problems.
- If you are supposed to skip a dose before having a test, talk to your doctor about how to do so. Also ask what you should do if you accidentally miss a dose.
- Write down the date you start or stop any medication or increase or decrease its dosage, and note any side effects or changes to your health or mood. Inform your doctor about anything you notice.

High Blood Pressure

If your blood pressure consistently measures 140/90 or greater, you've got hypertension, or high blood pressure. (See Chapter 3 for more information about blood pressure and what these numbers mean.) The force of blood pushing against the walls of your arteries as your heart pumps blood through the circulatory system is too strong, and it could damage the arterial lining. Over time, high blood pressure can lead to atherosclerosis—the stiffening of arteries and buildup of plaque deposits that sets the stage for heart disease—as well as to other health problems such as stroke, kidney disease, or blindness.

You're also at risk if your blood pressure isn't quite that high. Doctors define the range of values between 120/80 and 140/90 as "prehypertension," a condition that often leads to full-blown hypertension. About 59 million Americans fit into this category. Even if their blood pressure never increases into the hypertensive range, they still run a much higher risk of heart attack and other problems related to atherosclerosis than do people with normal blood pressure—that is, anything at or below 120/80. (Very low blood pressure can be a problem, but generally the lower the values are, the better.) A study published in 2005 found that people with prehypertension are nearly twice as likely to have heart disease, and more than three times as likely to suffer heart attacks, as "normotensive" individuals.

> People in their 50s who have normal blood pressure live five years longer, on average, than people with high blood pressure.

Hypertension's toll

Hypertension is sometimes called the "silent killer" because it usually comes with no symptoms. People with hypertension usually feel fine, making the condition a double-edged sword: Often it remains undiagnosed, but even those who know they have it must be rigorous about keeping up their course of treatment.

For a better idea of hypertension's dangers, consider these facts:

- The World Health Organization has estimated that hypertension causes 1 in every 8 deaths worldwide, making it the planet's third leading killer.
- Hypertension is a primary or contributing cause in more than 10 percent of deaths in the United States each year.
- Of the 50 million Americans with hypertension, 32 percent are unaware they have the condition; only 27 percent receive treatment that restores their blood pressure to normal; 26 percent receive inadequate treatment and fail to control their blood pressure; and 15 percent receive no treatment at all.
- Efforts to manage high blood pressure account for 1 in 6 office visits to health care providers.
- Data from the Framingham Heart Study suggest that people whose blood pressure is normal at age 55 have a 90 percent likelihood of developing hypertension within their lifetimes.

Wanted: better control of hypertension

Both hypertension and prehypertension call for treatment. Exercise, weight loss, and stress reduction often do the trick; in other cases, though, additional treatment with one or more antihypertensive drugs may be necessary.

Despite the existence of effective treatments, many people with blood-pressure problems fail to control the condition. There are three main reasons this is so:

1. Because high blood pressure is almost always asymptomatic—that is, causing no symptoms—people who have it may feel fine and therefore may not maintain their treatment regimen.

2. All antihypertensive drugs cause side effects, prompting some people to stop taking them. If your medication is causing unpleasant side effects, let your doctor know; a different treatment regimen will often control your blood pressure with less-vexing side effects.

3. People don't monitor their blood pressure closely after a treatment begins, thinking the problem is solved. Whenever you visit your doctor, ask that you have your blood pressure checked to see if your treatment is adequately controlling it. Or take your blood pressure yourself at the pharmacy, grocery store, or any other place that offers blood-pressure testing.

If you've begun antihypertensive therapy, close monitoring during the first months—and routinely after that—is vital. Not every medication works for everyone, and some lose effectiveness over time. Your doctor can solve the problem by increasing the dose, switching you to a new drug, or starting a combination of drugs. Don't be concerned if you need to take two or more drugs to keep your blood pressure in check: That may be the most effective plan for you.

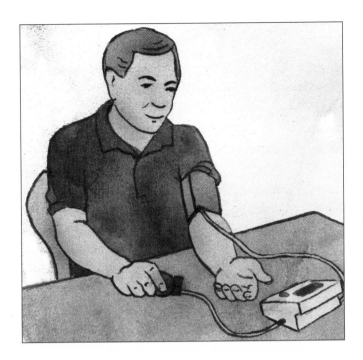

The Importance of Self-Monitoring

If you are about to start treatment for hypertension, one of the best things you can do for yourself is to invest in a home blood-pressure monitor. (The simple steps required to take your own blood pressure are described on pages 41–42.) If you monitor your blood pressure at least three times a week, you'll be able to track the positive results of your treatment—or alert your doctor if an adjustment is necessary. This in turn will help motivate you to stick with your antihypertensive therapy.

Antihypertensive Drugs

Five basic classes of antihypertensive medications—more than 100 different drugs—are commonly used to control high blood pressure. The best choice for you is whichever treatment achieves the desired blood-pressure goal with the fewest side effects; you may also need to take a specific type of antihypertensive drug if you have another illness such as diabetes.

The five classes of antihypertensive drugs are reviewed below. Tips on what to do before starting the medication (and once you're on it), as well as possible side effects, are included for the three most widely prescribed classes.

In 2003, the National Committee on Detection, Evaluation, and Treatment of High Blood Pressure recommended diuretics as the initial treatment of choice for hypertension.

Diuretics

These drugs, also known as "water pills," have been in use for more than 40 years. Diuretics treat fluid retention, which can cause swelling, weight gain, and shortness of breath, but they also help your body get rid of excess salt. Flushing sodium from blood-vessel walls allows those vessels to dilate, or expand, which reduces blood pressure.

Most patients tolerate diuretics very well and can continue taking them for many years without difficulty. Diuretics can help you feel better and have more energy. In addition to hypertension, diuretics are prescribed for heart failure, kidney problems, liver problems, and glaucoma.

Before you start a diuretic, tell your doctor or pharmacist if:

- You are taking any other medicine. This includes prescription and nonprescription drugs.
- You are taking herbal supplements.
- You have other medical problems or you are pregnant or breastfeeding.
- You have ever had an allergic reaction to any medicine or food.

TIPS FOR TAKING A DIURETIC

- Take your diuretic exactly as directed. If you have any questions, talk to your doctor or pharmacist.
- Most regimens call for taking a diuretic early in the day.
- If your treatment includes two or more doses a day, take the last one before dinner. That way, you'll get up fewer times during the night to urinate.
- If you miss a dose, take it as soon as you remember. If it is almost time for the next dose, skip the missed dose. Do not take a double dose.

TIPS FOR SAFE USE OF DIURETICS

Weigh yourself at the same time on the same scale every morning, wearing the same clothes. Weigh yourself after urinating and before eating.

- A sudden weight gain or a steady rise in weight tells you that your body is retaining water and salt. Call your doctor if you notice a 3- to 5-pound weight gain in less than a week. You may need to adjust your dose.
- Follow your doctor's guidelines for limiting your salt intake.
- Follow any guidelines your doctor gives you for eating high-potassium foods. Diuretics can deplete the body's potassium reserves.
- Get up slowly when you are sitting or lying down. If a diuretic has lowered your blood pressure, you may become lightheaded if you rise too quickly.
- Refill your prescription before you would run out of medicine.
- Do not share your medicine with anyone.

POSSIBLE SIDE EFFECTS OF DIURETICS

Call your doctor right away if you have any of these side effects:

- Extreme tiredness or weakness
- Excessive thirst or a dry mouth
- Muscle cramps or joint pain
- Chest pains or changes in heartbeat
- Numbness or tingling in hands, feet, or lips
- Diarrhea, constipation, nausea, or vomiting
- Ringing in the ears
- Lightheadedness when getting up after sitting or lying down
- Skin rash
- Headache, blurred vision, or confusion
- Rapid or excessive weight gain
- Loss of appetite
- Depression or sadness
- Shortness of breath or difficulty in breathing or swallowing
- Impotence

Beta blockers

Beta blockers, which lower blood pressure by slowing the heart and reducing the force with which it pumps blood through the circulatory system, have been in use for about 35 years. They also reduce your heart's workload and help it beat more regularly. In addition to lowering blood pressure, beta blockers may ease chest pain if you have angina. They can also reduce your risk of another heart attack if you have already had one.

Before you start on a beta blocker, tell your doctor or pharmacist if:

- You are taking any other prescription or over-the-counter medicines. This includes vitamin supplements and herbal remedies.
- You have other health problems or you are pregnant or breastfeeding. Be sure to mention if you have asthma, chronic obstructive pulmonary disease, or diabetes. Beta blockers can complicate these conditions.
- You have had an allergic reaction to any medicine or food.

TIPS FOR TAKING A BETA BLOCKER

- Take your beta blocker exactly as directed. If you don't fully understand the directions on the label, ask your doctor or pharmacist to clarify them.
- Take your beta blocker at the same time or times each day.
- If you take a long-acting tablet or capsule, swallow it whole with a glass of water. Do not chew it, crush it, or break it open unless instructed that it's okay to do so.
- If you miss a dose, take it as soon as you remember—unless it's almost time for your next dose. Do not take a double dose.

TIPS FOR USING BETA BLOCKERS SAFELY

- Do not stop taking your beta blocker unless your doctor tells you to. Doing so can make your condition worse. When it is time to stop, follow your doctor's instructions.
- Do not drive or use heavy or dangerous machinery unless you are certain your beta blocker will not make you sleepy or dizzy.

- Talk to your doctor or pharmacist before you take any other medicines.
- Refill your prescription before you run out.
- Do not share your medicine with anyone.

POSSIBLE SIDE EFFECTS OF BETA BLOCKERS

Side effects may occur at first, but typically they disappear as your body adjusts to the medication. Call your doctor or pharmacist if these side effects bother you or persist:

- Dizziness or lightheadedness
- Tiredness, drowsiness, or weakness
- Impotence
- Trouble sleeping
- Depression
- Cold feeling in arms or legs

Call your doctor *right away* if you have any of these side effects:

- Wheezing or trouble breathing
- Chest pain or slowed or irregular heartbeat
- Swelling in the lower legs or feet
- Yellow skin or eyes
- Numbness or tingling
- Skin rash or itching

ACE inhibitors

Angiotensin-converting enzyme (ACE) inhibitors relax blood vessels, thus reducing blood pressure. They work by cutting the production of angiotensin I, which the body converts into angiotensin II, a hormone that constricts arteries. ACE inhibitors appear to be especially useful for hypertensive patients with diabetes.

Before you start taking an ACE inhibitor, tell your doctor or pharmacist if:

- You are taking any other prescription or over-the-counter medicines. This includes vitamin supplements and herbal remedies.

- You have other medical problems or you are pregnant or breastfeeding.
- You have ever had an allergic reaction to any medicine or food.

TIPS FOR TAKING AN ACE INHIBITOR

- Take your ACE inhibitor exactly as directed. If you have any questions, refer to the pharmacy leaflet that came with your medicine, or talk to your doctor or pharmacist.
- Do not change the dose or stop taking your medicine unless your doctor tells you to.
- If your doctor has told you to take your blood pressure, measure it as often as directed. Record the number each time.
- If you miss a dose, take it as soon as you remember—unless it's almost time for your next dose. If so, skip the missed dose. Do not take a double dose.

TIPS FOR USING ACE INHIBITORS SAFELY

- Make sure all your health care providers, including your dentist, know which ACE inhibitor you take. Some ACE inhibitors can interact with other medicines, including dental medications.
- Talk to your doctor about whether you can use a salt substitute or drink alcohol.
- Don't drive or stand up quickly if your medicine makes you dizzy or lightheaded.
- Refill your prescription before you would run out.
- Do not share your medicine with anyone.

POSSIBLE SIDE EFFECTS OF ACE INHIBITORS

Call your doctor right away if you have any of these side effects:

- A dry cough that is sporadic and doesn't go away (occurs in 4 to 10 percent of the population, more commonly in women)
- Swelling or a rash anywhere on the body
- Trouble breathing or swallowing

- Dizziness or lightheadedness
- Pain in joints
- Metallic or salty taste in the mouth, or decreased ability to taste
- Worsening of psoriasis

Angiotensin Receptor Blockers (ARBs)

ARBs block the action of angiotensin II, a hormone that constricts arteries. These drugs are especially for patients who experience side effects—a cough or rash, for example—when taking the more commonly prescribed ACE inhibitors. Talk with your doctor about how to take this medication and what to expect.

Calcium-channel blockers

Like other antihypertensive drugs, calcium-channel blockers work by relaxing blood vessels. They prevent calcium atoms from entering the heart muscle or the walls of blood vessels, which widens the blood vessels, decreasing blood pressure and making it easier for the heart to pump blood. There are two types of calcium-channel blockers—short-acting and long-acting. Heart-disease patients may need to use certain classes of short-acting calcium-channel blockers in combination with a beta blocker. Calcium blockers can produce leg swelling, particularly in women. Discuss other possible side effects with your doctor.

The Need to Mix & Match

Only about 40 to 50 percent of people with hypertension can lower their blood pressure into a safe range with one medication alone. More and more, doctors are treating patients with combinations of antihypertensive drugs from two or more classes. Some medications contain two antihypertension drugs in the same pill. Capozide® and Lotensin® HCT, for example—both available as generics—combine a diuretic with an ACE inhibitor. The ideal treatment for many patients blends low doses of two or more drugs, an approach that helps reduce the possibility of troubling side effects.

Finding the best hypertension treatment regimen may take a sustained effort—on your part and your doctor's. Don't be surprised, then, if your doctor switches your medication—or your dosage—several times over the first few months of treatment. Be patient, and work with your doctor by tracking your own blood pressure, following through with any required laboratory tests, and noting any troublesome side effects. Making the effort to lower elevated blood pressure is well worth it: Reducing blood pressure dramatically reduces the risk of dying from a heart attack or stroke. Bringing down your blood pressure also helps ward off enlargement of the heart and heart failure and helps prevent kidney disease.

High Cholesterol

Cholesterol is a naturally occurring type of fat (lipid) in your body that is a key component of cell membranes and a vital ingredient in the formation of testosterone, estrogen, and other hormones. But having too much total cholesterol—in particular, too much low-density lipoprotein (LDL, or "bad" cholesterol), or too little high-density lipoprotein (HDL, or "good" cholesterol)—in your blood can greatly increase your risk of having a heart attack or stroke. Indeed, cholesterol problems are one of the major risk factors for heart disease.

Cholesterol is the main substance found in atherosclerotic plaques, which are especially dangerous when they restrict blood flow in the brain (risk of stroke) and coronary arteries (risk of heart attack). The probability of plaque forming in your arteries becomes greater if the level of cholesterol in your bloodstream (often referred to as serum cholesterol) is abnormally high.

Not surprisingly, many studies have shown that the risk of dying from coronary artery disease (CAD) increases as cholesterol levels rise. One such study, the Multiple Risk Factor Intervention Trial, measured the total cholesterol levels of more than 360,000 middle-aged men and then followed them for six years. At the end of that time, men with total cholesterol levels above 300 mg/dL (milligrams per deciliter) were nearly four times more likely to have died from CAD than men whose cholesterol levels were below 180 mg/dL.

Cholesterol Numbers Explained

Your health care provider can measure your cholesterol levels with a simple blood test. The results indicate your total cholesterol level and also provide the numbers for your LDL and HDL cholesterol as well as other fats in the bloodstream. In general, your total cholesterol should be less than 200 mg/dL.

> Roughly 55 percent of American adults have total cholesterol levels higher than 200 mg/dL.

LDL is called "bad" cholesterol because it stays in the blood and contributes to plaque buildup on the insides of artery walls. People with heart disease or diabetes should have an LDL cholesterol level of 70 mg/dL or less.

HDL is called "good" cholesterol because it helps remove cholesterol from the bloodstream and delivers it to the liver for elimination from the body. HDL should be 40 mg/dL or higher for men, 50 mg/dL or higher for women.

Triglycerides are the main type of fat found in the body and in the diet. Triglyceride levels should be less than 150 mg/dL. (See Chapter 3 for more information about cholesterol.)

The Benefits of Drug Therapy

Clinical studies indicate that lowering the levels of LDL cholesterol in your bloodstream can sharply reduce your risk of having a heart attack. Lifestyle changes such as increasing exercise and observing a diet low in saturated fats and trans fats—an especially pernicious form of fat found in many processed foods—can help improve cholesterol levels. But when these measures don't suffice, cholesterol-lowering drugs can bring cholesterol to safe levels and significantly reduce the risk of a heart attack.

The most widely used cholesterol-lowering drugs are known as statins. These medicines do their work by blocking a certain enzyme from stimulating the production of cholesterol in the liver. This enzyme helps convert dietary fat into cholesterol for the body's use, but various factors—including a high-fat diet or a genetic predisposition—can make the liver produce too much cholesterol.

The statins' ability to block this enzyme has two important effects: The amount of cholesterol that the liver pours into the bloodstream decreases, and the amount of LDL cholesterol that the liver removes from the blood increases. (As a bonus, statins also lower triglyceride levels.)

Statin drugs can lower LDL cholesterol anywhere from 20 to 60 percent. (Generally speaking, each 10 percent drop in LDL cholesterol level lowers heart-attack risk by 20 percent.) Statins can also raise HDL cholesterol 2 to 10 percent. Several large clinical trials of statins have shown that statins can reduce both the number of deaths and the incidence of major cardiovascular events—including heart attacks, strokes, and angina—by as much as 20 to 30 percent.

Statins seem to have a favorable impact on the plaque that may have collected in arteries from atherosclerosis. Evidence indicates that statins stabilize these plaques and make them less likely to rupture (ruptured plaques can block blood flow and cause heart attacks and strokes). Some statins may even help shrink the size of plaque deposits.

Seven statin drugs are now on the market. Listed here by generic name (with the brand name in parentheses), they are: atorvastatin (Lipitor®), fluvastatin (Lescol®), lovastatin (Mevacor®), pravastatin (Pravachol®), rosuvastatin (Crestor®), simvastatin (Zocor®), and ezetimibe/simvastatin (Vytorin®). (Note: As of late 2006, generics were on the market only for Mevacor®, Pravachol®, and Zocor®.)

Statins are relatively safe, but their side effects can include constipation or diarrhea, dizziness or headache, gas or heartburn, nausea, and insomnia. Rarer but more serious side effects include fever, tiredness, or weakness; ongoing muscle aches, cramps, or tenderness; blurred vision; and skin rash or itching. Report any muscle pain or weakness or change in urine color to your health provider.

Because statins affect liver function, when they were first introduced there was much concern that they would damage the liver or worsen problems in patients with liver abnormalities. These fears have generally proved to be unfounded.

However, ask your doctor if any regular monitoring tests are needed to check how a certain medicine is working. Keep all laboratory appointments, and make sure your doctor knows your test results before she or he changes your treatment plan.

It's also critical for all statin users to have periodic blood tests to assess liver function. And if you drink alcohol or have active or chronic liver disease, it's best to avoid statins. Talk with your doctor about other choices.

Is It Too Late to Start?

If you've already suffered a heart attack or have been diagnosed with heart disease, you may assume it's too late for cholesterol-lowering medicines to help you very much—but think again.

Treating cholesterol problems not only helps prevent atherosclerosis but also seems to keep existing heart disease from getting worse; it may even reverse atherosclerosis by helping to dispel artery-clogging plaques. Improvements in cholesterol numbers actually benefit heart-disease patients more than otherwise healthy individuals with high cholesterol. That's at least partly because people who have previously had a heart attack, who have angina, or who have had angioplasty or coronary artery bypass graft surgery are five to seven times more likely than others to have another heart attack or require another medical procedure.

One study—the PROVE-IT trial, published in 2004—found that aggressively lowering LDL cholesterol levels in people who had recently suffered a heart attack significantly decreased their risk of a subsequent heart attack or other adverse event.

> The National Cholesterol Education Program recommends that all adults over 20 get a blood test to measure their total cholesterol level.

The treatment goal for healthy people with elevated LDL cholesterol is 100 mg/dL, but for heart-disease patients the goal is even lower. The 2004 update of the National Cholesterol Education Program guidelines urged doctors to reduce their heart-disease patients' LDL cholesterol levels to 70 mg/dL or even lower.

Despite overwhelming evidence that cholesterol-lowering therapy can help, countless heart-disease patients are not benefiting: Either their doctors have not prescribed medication, or the patients (for reasons of cost or side effects) do not take the drugs prescribed for them. If you have heart disease or have previously had a heart attack or stroke and are not currently taking a cholesterol-lowering drug, talk to your doctor about getting your cholesterol levels checked—and, if necessary, getting started on a statin or other cholesterol-lowering drug.

Other Classes of Cholesterol-Lowering Drugs

The statins are the leading class of cholesterol-lowering drugs because of their superior ability to reduce total and LDL cholesterol levels and because of patients' relative tolerance of their side effects. Several other drug classes, described below, may be more appropriate in certain circumstances.

Ezetimibe (Zetia)

This cholesterol-lowering drug, like the statins, reduces total and LDL cholesterol, but it does so by restricting the small intestine's absorption of dietary cholesterol rather than by decreasing the liver's production of cholesterol. Zetia® can serve as an alternative for people who can't tolerate statins; it is also prescribed for those unable to control their cholesterol by diet alone.

Because Zetia® and the statins work differently, doctors sometimes prescribe them together (unless the patient has liver disease) to maximize cholesterol reduction.

Fibrates (fibric acid derivatives)

This class of drugs consists of gemfibrozil (Lopid®) and fenofibrate (TriCor®), which block the production of proteins that transport cholesterol in the bloodstream. Unlike the statins, fibrates have only modest effects against LDL cholesterol, but they are effective at reducing triglyceride levels. If your triglycerides are too high, your doctor may put you on one of the fibrates. They are generally well tolerated but can cause feelings of fullness, bloating, or heartburn after eating; dizziness; or changes in the sense of taste and touch.

Niacin

This B vitamin, also known as nicotinic acid, is found in small amounts in vitamin pills and is part of a healthy diet. At high doses—

Ways to Raise HDL Levels

High LDL ("bad" cholesterol) and low HDL ("good" cholesterol) are independent risk factors for heart disease. Statins can dramatically lower LDL levels, but they are notably less effective at raising levels of HDL, an equally important strategy. Fortunately, you can take a number of actions—none of which requires a prescription—to boost your HDL levels.

Start exercising: Among healthy but sedentary people, regular aerobic exercise can increase HDL cholesterol levels by 3 to 9 percent. The greatest increases in HDL occur with frequent low-intensity exercise, such as five 30-minute sessions per week. A boost in HDL levels may occur after as few as eight weeks of regular exercise. (Regrettably, walking appears to have little effect on HDL levels.)

Stop smoking: When people stop smoking, their HDL levels increase by an average of 4 mg/dL. This increase is usually more pronounced in women than in men.

Lose weight: The effects of weight loss on HDL levels are particularly pronounced in obese people who lose considerable amounts of weight. HDL levels increase by $\frac{1}{3}$ mg/dL for every 2.2 pounds of weight reduction. A reasonable weight-loss goal is one pound per week.

Drink alcohol in moderation (one or two drinks per day): Drinking 1 ounce of alcohol daily increases HDL cholesterol levels by an average of 4 milligrams per deciliter, regardless of the type of alcoholic beverage consumed. Numerous studies have concluded that, for middle-aged people, moderate alcohol consumption reduces the risk of heart attack by 30 to 50 percent. But if you have liver disease, heart failure due to alcohol, or are prone to alcoholism, the risks of alcohol clearly outweigh its benefits.

1 or 2 grams a day—niacin can control cholesterol in several ways: It can reduce total cholesterol by up to 25 percent, lower triglyceride levels, and raise HDL levels. Niacin is relatively inexpensive and widely available without a prescription, but it can cause a high number of side effects, including rashes, worsening of gout, and—especially early in therapy—facial flushing that lasts several minutes (and that many people find highly unpleasant). People with chronic liver disease, diabetes, or peptic ulcer should not take niacin.

Dietary fiber

Technically it's not a drug, but dietary fiber—particularly soluble fiber—can help lower cholesterol levels. Oat bran, a good source of soluble fiber, gained fame a few years ago when studies showed that it could help lower cholesterol levels. Similar results can also be obtained with other foods high in soluble fiber, such as beans, barley, peas, and apple pulp.

Supplementing one's diet with psyllium, a soluble fiber derived from the husks of psyllium seeds, can yield a 15 percent reduction in LDL cholesterol levels, reports the American Heart Association. (NIH-sponsored research, by contrast, found psyllium to be neither safe nor effective; see warning box, page 202.) Psyllium is the primary ingredient in several widely available fiber-based laxatives. If you are taking an oral medication, you should take a fiber-based laxative at least two hours before or two hours after taking the medication so as not to interfere with that drug's effectiveness.

Treating Angina

The pain of an angina attack is the body's way of indicating that the heart muscle isn't getting enough oxygen, usually because atherosclerotic plaque deposits have narrowed one or more coronary arteries and restricted blood flow to heart tissue. Angina is thus one of the most important symptoms of coronary artery disease (CAD)— and a clear indication that you need to seek treatment.

Angina symptoms vary from individual to individual. The classic signs are pain, heaviness, tightness, pressure, or aching in the chest; these sensations can also occur in the back, neck, throat, or jaw, as well as the shoulders, arms, elbows, or wrists. Angina may also be accompanied by tiredness, nausea, sweating, shortness of breath, lightheadedness, and increased or irregular heartbeat. Sometimes the symptoms are less clear-cut and may only be identifiable if you've already been told you have angina and know what to expect.

When attacks occur is a key indicator of how advanced the underlying heart disease is. So-called stable angina strikes predictably,

Aspirin: The "Forgotten" Wonder Drug?

Few medicine cabinets are without it, and more and people are aware of its powerful ability to treat and even prevent some of the complications of heart disease. Surprisingly, though, aspirin remains in certain ways a "forgotten" drug for treating cardiovascular problems.

Because aspirin inhibits the formation of blood clots that can trigger heart attacks and strokes, clinical guidelines recommend it as a daily preventive treatment for people with heart disease and other conditions related to atherosclerosis—especially those who have already had a heart attack or stroke. Some protocols even suggest a daily "baby" aspirin (81 mg) for men over 50 and women over 60 who have just one of the risk factors for heart disease.

A 2005 study found, however, that only about a third of those who could benefit are routinely following so-called aspirin therapy. In high-risk patients, aspirin may be just as effective as cholesterol-lowering statins at reducing the chances of a heart attack or other cardiovascular problem, yet doctors seem to rely on the more expensive prescription medication more often.

If you've had a heart attack or stroke or been diagnosed with heart disease, talk with your doctor about whether aspirin therapy might be right for you. (Regular doses of aspirin can cause serious gastrointestinal bleeding in some patients, so don't start a daily regimen on your own without consulting your doctor.) And always have at least a couple of full-strength (325 mg) aspirins available at all times, even when you're out: Research indicates that taking an aspirin right after a heart attack or stroke might actually save your life.

during exertion or in upsetting or tense situations. Unstable angina can occur at any time, even at rest, and is very much of a red flag that atherosclerosis has developed to a dangerous degree, and that the risk of heart attack or stroke is great. (For more information on angina, see Chapter 4.)

See your doctor as soon as possible if you think you've had an angina attack or if existing angina has grown worse or less predictable. You may be able to control it with lifestyle changes if it's mild. More serious cases of angina—indicating more advanced heart disease—usually call for treatment with medication or perhaps even a medical procedure to clear or bypass clogged arteries. The sections immediately below describe the standard forms of drug therapy for angina. See pages 175–190 for information about medical procedures to treat the restricted blood flow through coronary arteries that causes angina.

Taking Nitroglycerin

One drug frequently chosen to treat angina is nitroglycerin. It widens blood vessels, allowing blood to reach the heart muscle more efficiently and supply it with the oxygen it needs. Nitroglycerin comes in two forms: one to stop an attack in progress and the other to prevent attacks from recurring.

Because both forms of nitroglycerin are especially powerful medications, it's crucial to take it exactly as directed by your doctor. Above all else, never take more or less than the prescribed dose.

Stopping an Angina Attack with Fast-acting Nitroglycerin

Fast-acting nitroglycerin products, which come in spray or tablet form, stop angina attacks that are already under way. Carry your fast-acting tablets or spray with you at all times.

If you use fast-acting tablets and feel angina:

- Sit down (you may become dizzy).
- Place one tablet under your tongue (sublingual administration). Or place it between your lip and gum, or between your cheek and gum (buccal administration).
- Let the tablet dissolve completely; do not chew or swallow it. Do not eat, drink, smoke, or chew tobacco while the tablet is dissolving.

If you use a fast-acting spray and feel angina:

- Sit down (you may become dizzy).
- Hold the sprayer right in front of your mouth.
- Spray once under your tongue or inside your cheek. Do not inhale.
- Close your mouth. Wait a few seconds before you swallow.

Whether you use tablets or a spray, take only one dose, then sit quietly for five minutes.

- If the angina goes away, you should rest a while before resuming your normal routine.
- If the angina does not go away or gets worse, call 911 immediately. Do not delay—you may be having a heart attack!

Preventing angina with long-acting nitroglycerin

Long-acting nitroglycerin prevents angina attacks from recurring. It's available as patches, tablets, capsules, or ointments. The directions for use vary with each type.

Patch. Apply a new patch every morning. Leave it on for as long as your doctor instructs, then remove it. Find a new place for each day's patch, but avoid areas that are hairy, cut, irritated, scarred, or tattooed.

Tablet or capsule. Take the tablet or capsule one hour before eating or two hours afterward. Swallow it with a full glass of water. Do not break, chew, or crush the tablet or capsule.

Ointment. Squeeze the prescribed amount of ointment onto the measuring paper that came with the tube. Use the paper to spread a thin, even layer on a clean patch of skin; do not rub it in. Tape the paper in place with skin tape for as long as directed, then remove it. Use a new area of skin for each application.

PRECAUTIONS

Tell your health care provider about other prescription and nonprescription drugs and dietary supplements you are taking. Nitroglycerin interacts with certain other medications to significantly lower blood pressure and cause dizziness, lightheadedness, or fainting.

In particular, never take the erectile dysfunction drugs Viagra®, Levitra®, or Cialis® if you have used a short-acting nitroglycerin recently or if you are on a long-acting nitroglycerin all the time. This is a dangerous combination; it can be fatal.

Do not suddenly stop using a long-acting nitroglycerin. Doing so could bring on angina. Check with your health care provider before stopping this medication for any reason.

Limit alcohol. Drinking too much alcohol while on nitroglycerin therapy can cause dizziness or fainting.

Check the expiration date. Nitroglycerin loses its effectiveness over time.

Call your health care provider right away if you experience:

• Chest pain that lasts longer, is more severe, or happens more often than is typical for your angina
• An irregular or changed heartbeat
• Shortness of breath
• Blurred vision or a severe headache

Treatment for a Heart Attack

Heart attacks occur most often when plaque in the wall of a coronary artery ruptures, which causes a blood clot to form. If the clot completely obstructs the artery, a part of the heart muscle is deprived of oxygen. That area of heart muscle will be irreversibly damaged unless blood flow is restored within 30 minutes or a few hours at most. This region of dead tissue can no longer contribute to the heart's overall pumping action.

Time is therefore very much of the essence. The sooner you get treatment, the better your chances of avoiding tissue death and permanent damage to the heart. This in turn is why it's so crucially important to get to a hospital at the first sign of a heart attack. And if possible, take a 325 mg aspirin right away; a natural blood thinner, it can help blood flow through severely clogged arteries.

It bears repeating: Prompt therapy can minimize heart-muscle death.

Clot-Dissolving Drugs

Restoring blood flow is the No. 1 priority in treating a heart attack. When you arrive at the hospital, emergency-room personnel will most likely administer thrombolytic drugs—that is, drugs that dissolve blood clots immediately. Thrombolytic drugs (including streptokinase, urokinase, anistreplase, and tissue plasminogen activator, or TPA or TNKase) are injected directly into your bloodstream.

Recognize the Signs

Heart attacks typically cause severe pain, but there are other indications as well. Don't ignore any of the signs of a heart attack, which include:

- Pain or discomfort in the chest or in the jaw, abdomen, arm, or neck. The pain may be extreme, crushing, burning, or squeezing, and it may radiate from the chest down one or both arms.
- Nausea or vomiting
- Weakness or lightheadedness
- Shortness of breath
- Anxiety or a feeling of doom

If you experience any of these signs:

- Don't ignore them or tell yourself they'll go away.
- Call 911 or your local emergency number.
- Stay calm.
- Take nitroglycerin if you have your own prescription for it.
- Wait for help to arrive. (Unlock your door if you can.)
- Rest in a comfortable position.
- Loosen tight clothing.
- Don't drive yourself to the hospital.
- Take an aspirin tablet. Taking an aspirin within 24 hours of having a heart attack reduces the risk of dying by 23 percent.

Thrombolytic drug therapy restores blood flow to heart-muscle cells in about 80 percent of heart-attack patients who receive treatment within two hours of the onset of heart-attack symptoms. Little or no tissue death occurs, thus preserving more of the heart's pumping ability. Drug therapy that begins more than two hours after the first sign of symptoms achieves much more modest results. Some tissue death may be prevented, but irreversible damage almost always occurs, and is often fatal.

Emergency Angioplasty

In some cases, the best treatment for a heart attack may be an emergency medical procedure. Angioplasty, one of the most effective techniques for clearing clogged coronary arteries, can be performed

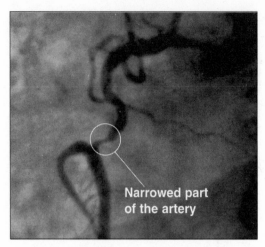

> Angiogram showing a constricted artery.

on an emergency basis at some medical centers. Clinical trials have found that it works at least as well as clot-dissolving drugs to restore blood flow to damaged tissue after a heart attack, and it's particularly valuable as an alternative to thrombolytic medications in patients who have gone into shock or developed very low blood pressure after an attack. See pages 177–181 for more information about angioplasty.

Finding & Treating Artery Blockages

When a diagnostic evaluation of your risk factors, your symptoms, and your medical history leads your doctor to believe that your coronary arteries may be narrowed by plaque, further testing can pinpoint any blockages. A cardiologist or other specialist can then employ any of several medical procedures to solve the problem. Sometimes locating and widening a narrowed artery are part of the same procedure.

Pinpointing blocked arteries

A two-stage medical procedure helps specialists locate narrowed or blocked coronary arteries. During cardiac catheterization (or cardiac cath), a thin, flexible tube inserted through a blood vessel in the arm, wrist, or groin is threaded into the heart. Once the catheter is in place, x-ray dye (contrast) is injected through it. (You may feel a warm flush

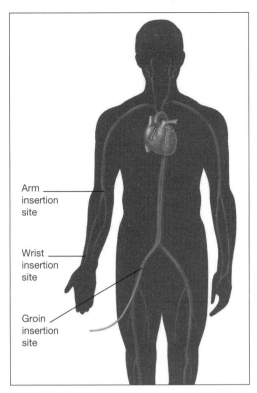

Arm
insertion
site

Wrist
insertion
site

Groin
insertion
site

> Possible insertion sites

as this happens.) The dye flows through the heart's arteries, creating an image on a special kind of x-ray called an angiogram. This procedure, known as coronary angiography, shows the coronary arteries in detail, revealing the precise location of any blockages.

Widening affected arteries

If an angiogram shows a narrowing or blockage, your doctor may choose balloon angioplasty or stenting to widen the affected arteries. Both of these procedures are done in the catheterization laboratory, either right after coronary angiography or later, after further evaluation. Depending on the nature and size of the blockage, balloon angioplasty may suffice, or it may be supplemented with stenting.

BALLOON ANGIOPLASTY TO WIDEN ARTERIES

Balloon angioplasty works best when the narrowing involves a small region of a single artery. Blockages that are more extensive—or

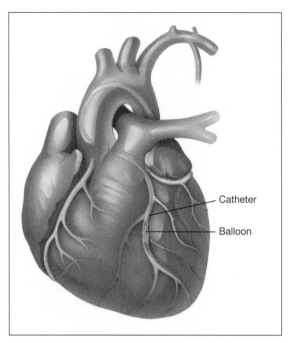

Catheter

Balloon

> A balloon-tipped catheter in place.

those in regions difficult to reach with a catheter—may require coronary artery bypass surgery. (See pages 183–190).

The technique is relatively simple to describe. A catheter tipped with a small, deflated "balloon" is threaded to the targeted site; the balloon is then inflated to widen the artery. It's also a relatively painless procedure: You'll be awake during balloon angioplasty, but you'll be given medication to help you relax.

Inserting the catheter and moving the balloon to the proper position involves several steps. First, a sheath is inserted into an artery near the surface of your skin at one of several possible locations, such as your wrist or groin. Next, a guiding catheter is inserted through the sheath and gently fed to the narrowed part of the artery. A guide wire is then inserted through the guiding catheter and moved to the same location. The doctor tracks the movement of the guide wire on a video monitor. Finally, a balloon-tipped catheter is inserted through the guiding catheter and threaded over the guide wire until it reaches the targeted spot.

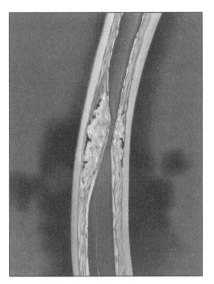

The guide wire is positioned.

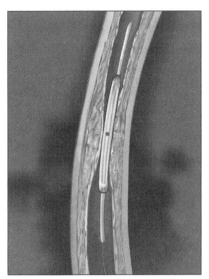

The balloon-tipped catheter reaches the narrowing.

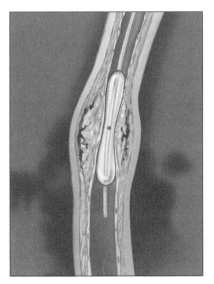

The balloon is inflated.

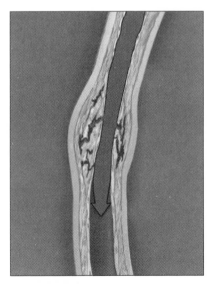

Blood flow improves.

> How balloon angioplasty works

When to Call Your Doctor

C all your doctor if you notice any of the following after your angioplasty procedure:

- Angina
- A fever above 100° F (37.8° C)
- Pain, swelling, redness, bleeding, or drainage at the insertion site
- Blood in your urine, black or tarry stools, or any other bleeding
- Severe pain, coldness, or a bluish color in the leg or arm where the sheath was inserted

Once the balloon-tipped catheter is in the proper position, the balloon is inflated and deflated one or more times. Each inflation increases the artery's diameter by compressing the plaque and stretching the artery wall. You may feel chest pain when the balloon is inflated—a result of blood flow being briefly blocked off to an area of your heart. Tell the doctor if you do so the balloon can be quickly deflated.

An angiogram is taken to make sure the artery has been opened and blood flow has improved. The balloon is then deflated, and the catheters and guide wire are removed. With the artery now open, blood flows freely to the heart muscle.

Recovering from angioplasty

After angioplasty, you will be taken to a cardiac care unit, a special recovery room, or your hospital room. For a few hours you'll remain on a heart monitor and have an intravenous (IV) line. Your pulse, blood pressure, and insertion site will be checked often. The sheath may remain in place for several hours. If the insertion site was in the groin, you may need to lie down and keep your leg still for several hours after the sheath is removed.

If there are no problems, you will most likely go home the day after the procedure. You'll be told about medications, follow-up care, and follow-up visits.

In the vast majority of cases, angioplasty succeeds in keeping a once-narrowed artery open for at least a year—and often much longer. In 10 to 20 percent of patients, though, the artery narrows again in less than a year, a problem known as restenosis. A second angioplasty may solve the problem, or stenting can provide a more permanent solution.

Stenting

A stent is a tiny, flexible, wire-mesh tube that your doctor positions in a narrowed or blocked coronary artery. It stays in place permanently. Many patients who undergo balloon angioplasty are candidates for stents, which help to prevent coronary arteries from renarrowing.

The procedure for positioning a stent is the same as for balloon angioplasty. A balloon-tipped catheter with a collapsed stent mounted over the tip is threaded to the narrowed part of the artery, and the balloon is inflated. This pushes plaque against the artery wall. It also opens the stent. The balloon is then deflated and removed, leaving the stent in place. If the narrowed portion of the artery is large enough, more than one stent may be deployed.

DRUG-ELUTING STENTS

Some stents are "drug-eluting," meaning they release medication slowly over time. The medication helps to minimize the amount of scar tissue that forms inside the artery. Drug-eluting stents tend to be more effective at preventing restenosis in healthier patients.

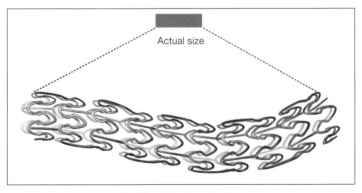

Actual size

> Magnified view of stent

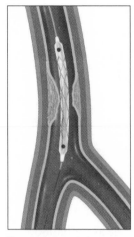 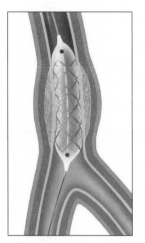 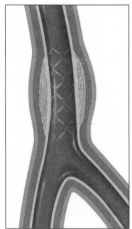

| The stent, mounted on a balloon, is slid into place. | The balloon is inflated; this opens the stent. | The stent stays in place, holding the artery open and letting blood flow. |

> How stents work

Risks and complications

Cardiac cath, coronary angiography, angioplasty, and stenting all involve some degree of risk. The risk is higher, however, with angioplasty and stenting. Risks and possible complications include:

- Bleeding or clotting
- Tearing of the artery lining
- Abnormal heartbeat (arrhythmia)
- Allergic reaction to the x-ray dye
- Kidney damage or failure
- The need for emergency bypass surgery (very rare)
- Heart attack, stroke, or death (very rare)

Recovery

With all of the above procedures, you may need to keep still, with your leg or arm extended, for two to six hours—how long depends partly on where the catheter was inserted and how the site was closed. You'll be closely monitored after the procedure until you're ready to go home. You can go home when:

- Your condition appears stable.
- The insertion site is not bleeding.
- Your blood tests have been cleared by your doctor.
- You have no signs of infection.
- You can urinate.

If you had only an angiogram, you may be able to go home within eight hours, and possibly as early as an hour after the procedure. After angioplasty or stenting, you are likely to stay in the hospital overnight (you'll be given instructions for post-operative care). At follow-up visits, your doctor will assess your progress, checking for any residual symptoms to see if the treatment succeeded.

Coronary artery bypass grafting

Some artery blockages are too extensive to qualify for treatment with angioplasty or stenting; instead, they require coronary artery bypass graft (CABG) surgery. The purpose of CABG is to create a new pathway through which blood can flow, bypassing the blocked portion of an artery.

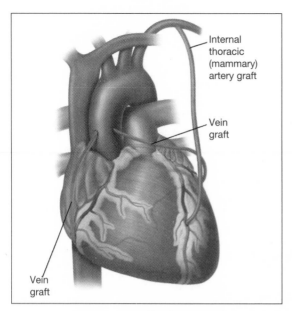
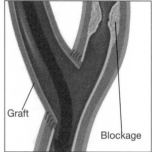

> How bypass grafts reroute blood flow

During CABG surgery, part of a healthy blood vessel is taken from the leg or elsewhere in the body; sometimes a vessel in the chest called the internal mammary artery is used. The bypass graft can reroute blood around the coronary-artery blockage in several different ways. A common CABG procedure involves connecting one end of a saphenous-vein segment (taken from the leg) to the aorta, close to where the coronary arteries normally originate; the other end of the segment is connected to the diseased coronary artery downstream from the blockage. Blood then flows through the graft, skirting the blocked section of the artery.

Knowing what to expect during bypass surgery can help ease your mind. Confidence that a team of skilled professionals is handling your surgery is vital, so grill them beforehand on their credentials and the number of times they perform your specific procedure in any given year. Ask your doctor to explain the risks of surgery and answer any questions you have.

A "PRE-CABG" CHECKLIST
- Your blood and urine may be tested for problems that could affect the surgery.

- You may meet with the anesthesiologist to discuss the medications that will keep you pain-free and unconscious during surgery. Insist on this meeting if you are fearful about anesthesia.
- Tell your doctor what medications, herbs, or supplements you're taking. This includes prescription and nonprescription medicines such as aspirin and other pain relievers. You may be asked to stop taking some of these before surgery.
- If you smoke, quit! Not smoking reduces the chance of lung problems as you recover from surgery.
- Don't eat or drink anything after midnight on the day before surgery; this includes water.

RISKS AND COMPLICATIONS OF BYPASS SURGERY

Your doctor will explain the possible risks of bypass surgery. These include:

- Excessive bleeding
- Infection of the incision sites
- Pneumonia (lung infection)
- Fast or irregular heartbeat
- Nerve injury or muscle spasms
- Breathing problems
- Memory problems or confusion
- Heart attack, stroke, or death

PREPARING THE BYPASS GRAFT

The first part of the surgery itself involves the "harvesting" of the bypass graft. If there is more than one blockage, the team will need more than one graft. Grafts are specifically chosen so as not to adversely affect blood flow in that part of the body.

REACHING THE HEART

While one surgeon on the bypass team retrieves the graft or grafts, another surgeon works to open the chest cavity. First, an incision is made down the middle of the chest. Then the breastbone (sternum) is surgically divided. The chest is then gradually pried open with special instruments called retractors so that the heart is accessible.

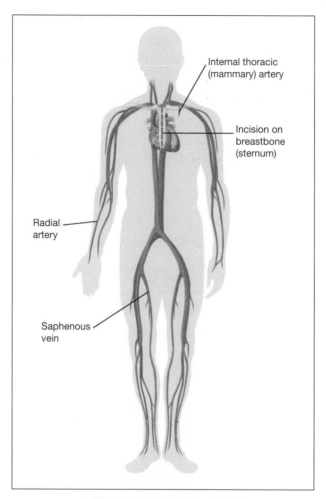

> Where bypass grafts are obtained

GOING "ON-PUMP"

Attaching grafts sometimes requires the surgical team to temporarily stop the heart. In these cases, the patient's blood circulates through a device called a heart-lung machine during surgery. As its name makes clear, this machine performs the functions of both the heart and the lungs, oxygenating the blood and pumping it through the circulatory system. This is known as an "on-pump" procedure. In other cases, the patient's heart is not stopped. These are known as "off-pump" or "beating-heart" procedures.

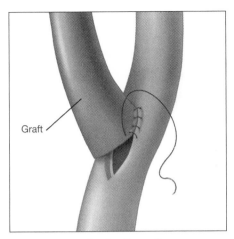

> Sewing the graft

ATTACHING THE GRAFT

A small opening is made in the diseased coronary artery below the blockage. If a saphenous vein or a radial artery (in the arm) is serving as the graft vessel, one end of the graft is sewn onto this opening; the other end is sewn onto the aorta. One advantage of using the internal thoracic (mammary) artery is that it is already attached to a branch of the aorta; for that reason, only one end needs to be sewn in place, on the coronary artery.

FINISHING UP THE CABG SURGERY

The breastbone is rejoined with wires that will stay in the chest permanently. The incision is closed and the patient is taken to the Intensive Care Unit (ICU) to begin recovery.

AFTER BYPASS SURGERY

When you wake up in the ICU, you will likely be thirsty, groggy, and cold. These sensations are common and temporary. ICU nurses are trained to anticipate your post-op needs.

A tube inserted through your mouth and into your throat will help you breathe at first. This is normal. You won't be able to talk with the tube in, but it will be removed as soon as you can breathe on your own. Then you will be asked to breathe deeply and cough frequently to keep your lungs clear.

You'll also be connected to tubes and machines that allow the ICU staff to monitor your health. One IV catheter in your wrist or neck will monitor blood and heart pressures; another IV supplies medications and fluids; and tubes drain fluid from your chest. The IV lines and tubes will be removed as your condition stabilizes.

Once you are stable, you will be moved to your hospital room. This may happen the same day as the surgery or a day or more later. Every patient recovers from bypass surgery at a different rate. Many people stay in the hospital for three to seven days. During this time, you'll have help getting out of bed and moving around. Doing so will improve blood flow and help you regain strength. Before you leave the hospital, your doctor will talk to you about the next steps of your recovery.

HEALING @ HOME

As with short-term post-operative recovery, every person's timetable for healing is different. But you should expect to wait about six to eight weeks before returning to your normal routine. During that time, be sure to keep in touch with your doctor and take your pre-scribed medications. Also, follow the instructions you've been given to help your body heal.

FOLLOW-UP CARE

To ensure a safe recovery, don't miss any follow-up visits with your doctor. You will likely get chest x-rays and take a treadmill stress test or other tests that will enable the doctor to evaluate your progress. Be sure that you continue to comply with instructions about how to care for your incision and ease back into daily activities. You may be referred to a cardiac rehabilitation program to help in your recovery.

Caring for your incision. For several weeks after surgery, your incision site may be bruised, itchy, numb, or sore. A few days after you go home, you can remove any loose strips of tape over the incision. Don't take a tub bath until your doctor says it is safe. A warm shower should be fine, but be aware you may feel weak the first few times you shower. Using a special shower chair can help.

Taking your medications. Your doctor may prescribe medications to reduce your blood pressure or increase your blood flow during the healing process. You may also be taking medications to lower your cholesterol or keep your blood from clotting. If you have questions, talk to your doctor or pharmacist. And keep the following tips in mind:

- Take your medications exactly as prescribed. Don't increase, decrease, or stop your medications without your doctor's okay.
- Ask about common side effects and what to do if you experience them.
- Tell your doctor if you get symptoms such as an upset stomach, vomiting, diarrhea, or a skin rash.
- Ask if any of your medications necessitate monitoring tests.
- Follow through with all necessary lab work.
- Ask your doctor before taking any over-the-counter medications.
- Keep an up-to-date list of all your medications. Include dosage and other instructions.

Walk your way to health. When you walk, your legs pump blood back to your heart, which improves overall blood flow. You may be asked to start with a five-minute walk three or four times a day. With your doctor's go-ahead, walk a little longer each day, slowly working up to 30 minutes a day. Check with your doctor before beginning any other exercise program.

Note: Leg swelling is common if a graft was taken from your leg. Frequent walks may help control the swelling.

RETURNING TO NORMAL LIFE
Ease your way back into routine activities. Here are some guidelines.

Household chores: Light housework, such as folding laundry or dusting, is okay after a few weeks. Wait at least six weeks before doing things that require pushing or pulling, such as mowing or vacuuming.

Driving: Let others drive for three to six weeks after your surgery. Steering can worsen the pain from your healing breastbone.

Lifting: Don't lift objects weighing more than five pounds until you're told it's okay; this includes grocery bags, briefcases, and many other objects. Heft a five-pound bag of flour or sugar if you need to gauge what's appropriate to lift. Don't be tempted even to hoist a small child onto your lap.

On the job: Follow your doctor's advice about returning to work. You may be able to resume a desk job in three or four weeks. If your work is more physically demanding, you may need to wait up to 12 weeks.

Making love: Unless your doctor advises otherwise, you can have sex as soon as you feel able. Try to avoid positions that put weight on your breastbone or upper arms. See Chapter 7 for more information on resuming intimacy.

Treating Heart Failure

When you have heart failure (sometimes called congestive heart failure), your heart does not pump blood as well as it should. This means that some parts of your body do not receive enough oxygen and don't function properly. Organs can be adversely affected, and heart failure can make it harder to do things that used to be easy, such as climbing stairs. A weakened or failing heart also causes blood to back up into the lungs and other parts of the body, inducing swelling (edema).

Heart failure is a chronic disease—it won't go away—but you can work with your health care provider to develop a treatment plan that will help you live longer and more comfortably.

What does heart failure feel like?

Here are some of the most common symptoms of heart failure. You may have many of these symptoms, or only a few.

- Shortness of breath, wheezing, or coughing when you exert yourself
- Weakness or tiredness with little effort
- Problems breathing when you're lying flat, or the need to sleep in a recliner or propped up on many pillows
- Waking up at night coughing or short of breath
- Rapid weight gain
- Swelling in the abdomen, ankles, or feet
- Confusion or trouble concentrating
- A racing or skipping heart
- Dizziness or fainting

THE TWO TYPES OF HEART FAILURE

Heart failure can happen in two ways. Systolic dysfunction means the heart has become weaker and doesn't pump enough blood to the lungs and the rest of the body when the ventricles contract. Diastolic dysfunction means the heart muscle has become stiff and is unable to relax between contractions, so that the ventricles don't fill with enough blood. In both types of heart failure, each heartbeat pumps less blood than it should. You may have one or both types of heart failure.

The amount of blood that pumps out of the heart with each beat is called the ejection fraction (EF). Although it's normal for some blood to stay in the ventricles after each heartbeat, during heart failure more blood stays in the chambers than normal, meaning less is "ejected" from the heart and sent to the rest of the body.

FLUID DYNAMICS

When the heart fails to pump enough blood, the body releases hormones to make the heart work harder. Some cause the heart muscle to grow larger; others tell it to pump faster. These compensations may work for a while, but the heart muscle cannot keep pace with these demands over the long term. In time, the extra work damages the heart even further.

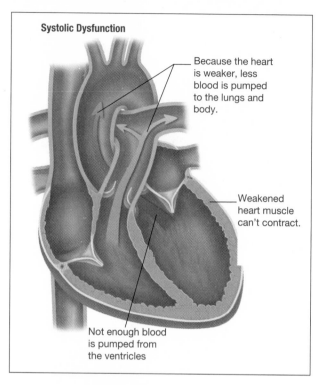

Systolic Dysfunction

Because the heart is weaker, less blood is pumped to the lungs and body.

Weakened heart muscle can't contract.

Not enough blood is pumped from the ventricles

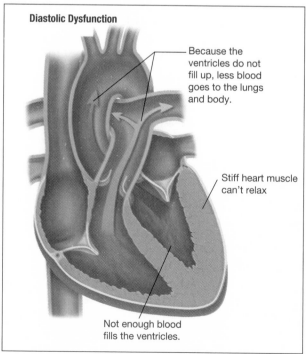

Diastolic Dysfunction

Because the ventricles do not fill up, less blood goes to the lungs and body.

Stiff heart muscle can't relax

Not enough blood fills the ventricles.

When heart failure starves your organs of adequate oxygen, they don't work properly, resulting in a range of problematic symptoms:

- The brain receives less oxygenated blood, making you feel confused or dizzy.
- The lungs fill with fluid, leaving you short of breath.
- The kidneys fail to rid the body of excess fluid, permitting it to back up in other parts of the body.
- Excess fluid may collect in the abdomen, ankles, and feet, causing edema (swelling).

Factors that cause heart failure

Heart failure can trace to any of several different health problems. Some of these damage the heart muscle so it cannot pump as well as it should. Others make the heart work too hard, weakening it by tiring it out.

HEART ATTACK

A heart attack—the most common cause of congestive heart failure—occurs when coronary artery disease blocks one or more coronary arteries. This stops blood flow to part of the heart muscle. Without oxygen-rich blood, the deprived part of the heart is permanently damaged and loses its ability to pump. The rest of the heart muscle must then work harder as a result. Over time, the strained heart muscle weakens and heart failure develops.

CAD

Coronary artery disease, or CAD, occurs when plaque deposits collect within the walls of the arteries. As plaque builds up, the arteries narrow, reducing blood flow to the heart muscle. Deprived of the oxygenated blood it needs to work normally, the muscle weakens—and heart failure develops.

HIGH BLOOD PRESSURE

High blood pressure (hypertension) occurs when blood pushes against artery walls harder than normal. Over time, this can cause

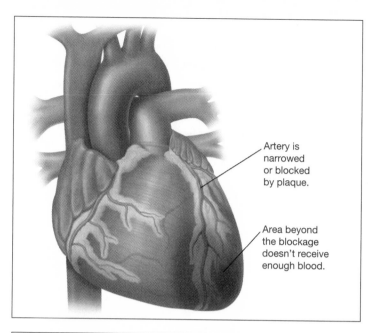

Artery is narrowed or blocked by plaque.

Area beyond the blockage doesn't receive enough blood.

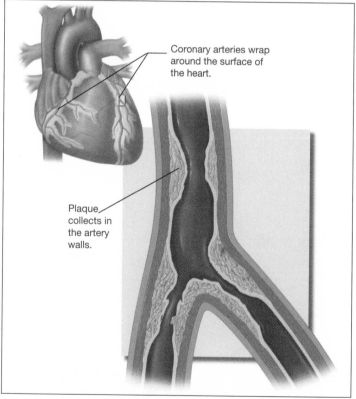

Coronary arteries wrap around the surface of the heart.

Plaque collects in the artery walls.

> How coronary artery disease affects your heart

the heart's chambers to enlarge. Failure to control high blood pressure eventually stretches and weakens the heart muscle and leads to heart failure.

VALVE DISEASE

Valve disease occurs when the valves between the chambers of the heart do not open or close properly. Healthy valves keep blood moving in the right direction. If a valve fails to open fully, the heart has to work harder to push blood through. If the valve fails to close tightly, blood leaks back into the chamber from which

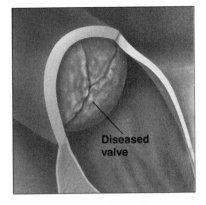

Diseased valve

it came, making the heart pump some of the same blood through the valve again. This extra work can weaken the heart and lead to heart failure.

CARDIOMYOPATHY

The tissue of the heart can itself become diseased, a condition known as cardiomyopathy. Among its causes are infections, alcohol abuse, and the toxic effects of certain drugs, including cocaine and cancer medications; cardiomyopathy can also be inherited. Cardiomyopathy causes the heart's chambers to enlarge and the heart muscle to stretch and weaken, leading to heart failure.

Health Problems That Influence Heart Failure

Certain other health problems can strain the heart and increase the probability that heart failure will develop. Diabetes makes CAD and heart failure more likely to occur. Chronic kidney problems can cause water retention, which means the heart has to pump more fluid and work harder.

A rapid or irregular heartbeat may occur along with heart failure; over time, this can worsen the problem. Heart failure is also more likely if you have severe anemia, an overactive thyroid gland, or congenital heart defects. Your doctor will explain whether any of these health problems may be contributing to your heart failure.

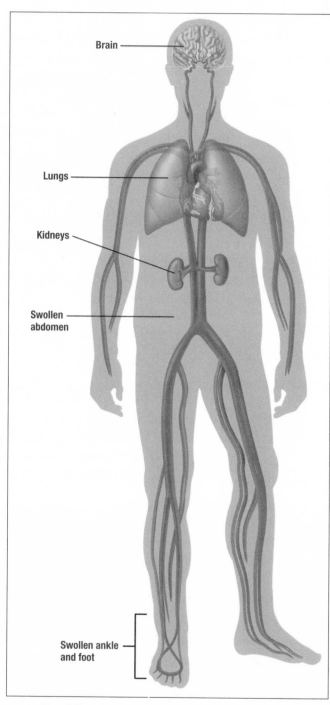

Brain

Lungs

Kidneys

Swollen
abdomen

Swollen ankle
and foot

> Heart failure affects organs and tissues throughout the body.

Changing Your Diet

Salt causes fluid to build up in the body and makes the heart work harder to pump blood. Fluid buildup from too much salt in the diet worsens the symptoms of heart failure, notably shortness of breath and edema (swelling). Controlling the amount of salt you eat may help prevent fluid from building up. Your doctor might also tell you to reduce the amount of fluid you drink.

READING FOOD LABELS

Read food labels to track how much sodium you consume. Remember that canned, frozen, and processed foods can be high in salt. Check the amount of sodium in each serving—and keep in mind that many packaged foods contain more than one serving! Also watch out for high-sodium ingredients such as MSG (monosodium glutamate), baking soda, and sodium phosphate. If you have heart failure, your health care provider will tell you how much sodium you can eat each day.

Nutrition Facts	
Serving size 1 cup	
Servings per container 2	

Amount Per Serving

Calories 90	Calories from fat 20
	% Daily Value
Total fat 2g	3%
Saturated fat 0g	
Trans fat 0g	
Cholesterol 10mg	3%
Sodium 890mg	39%
Total Carbohydrates 13g	4%
Dietary fiber 1g	4%
Sugars 1g	
Protein 6g	

Ingredients: Chicken broth, carrots, cooked white chicken meat (white chicken meat, water, salt, sodium phosphate, isolated soy protein, modified corn starch, corn starch), potatoes, celery, rice, monosodium glutamate. Contains soy.

LIMITING FLUIDS

You may need to limit your fluid intake to help prevent edema. "Fluid" includes anything that is liquid at room temperature, such as ice cream. If your doctor tells you to limit fluid, try these tips:

- Pour liquids into a measuring cup before you drink them. This will help you stay within your daily limits.
- Chill drinks to make them more refreshing.
- Suck on frozen lemon wedges to quench thirst.
- Drink only when you're thirsty.
- Rinse your mouth out with water, but don't swallow it.

• Chew sugarless gum or suck on hard candy to keep your mouth moist.

Heart-failure patients are also sometimes advised to restrict caffeine and alcohol; they may have to follow other dietary guidelines as well. If you have questions about what's safe to eat or drink, ask your health care provider.

Staying active to help your heart

Heart-failure patients benefit from staying active. Aerobic activities such as walking exercise the heart without straining it too much. When you remain active, you may also feel less tired, have fewer symptoms, and feel better about yourself and your health.

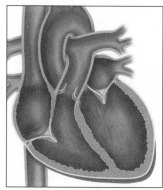

> The strong walls and clear gates of a healthy heart.

GOOD TO GO

Stay as active as feels comfortable. Continue day-to-day activities as long as you don't feel tired or short of breath. Try the following tips:

• Plan activities such as a walk around the block. If the weather is bad, walk inside a shopping mall instead. (Many hospitals sponsor mall-walking programs.) Light gardening and swimming are other options that may work for you. Talk to your health care provider about safe choices.
• Stop and rest if you feel tired or short of breath.
• Pace yourself: If you can't hold a conversation during an activity, you're pushing yourself too hard.
• Know your limits. You'll likely have good days and bad days.

Your health care provider can help you develop activity guidelines—perhaps even an exercise program—that works for you.

Medications to help with heart failure

Your health care provider will likely prescribe medications for heart failure and any underlying health problems. Certain medications

Signs of Overexertion

Stop exercising and call your doctor if you feel any of these symptoms:

- Chest pain or discomfort
- Burning, tightness, heaviness, or pressure in your chest
- Unusual aching in your arm, shoulders, neck, jaw, or back
- Trouble catching your breath
- A racing or skipping heart
- Extreme tiredness (especially after exercise)
- Lightheadedness, dizziness, or nausea

help you live longer by improving the way your heart pumps. Others relieve symptoms. Your doctor will work with you to find the best combination of medications.

Most heart-failure patients take several medications. The drugs you take will depend partly on the type of heart failure you have. Here are the most common ones:

- ACE inhibitors (see also pages 161–163) lower blood pressure and decrease strain on the heart; this makes it easier for the heart to pump. ACE inhibitors also block some of the hormones that the body releases to counter the effects of a weakened heart. One of these hormones, adrenaline, makes the heart beat faster and can damage the heart muscle. Angiotensin receptor blockers have similar effects and are sometimes prescribed instead of ACE inhibitors or along with them.
- Beta blockers (see also pages 160–161) help lower blood pressure and slow your heart rate; this reduces the amount of work your heart has to do. Beta blockers may improve the heart's pumping action over time.
- Hydralazine and nitrates improve heart function; in June 2005 the FDA approved their combined use (as BiDil) with ACE inhibitors and beta blockers in African Americans with heart failure. (African Americans are prone to heart failure that is particularly difficult to manage with drug therapy.)

M any heart medications cause side effects. These can include nausea, dry cough, dizziness, muscle cramps, or changes in your heart rhythm. Talk to your doctor or pharmacist to find out which side effects are most common for your medication. They can suggest ways to lessen any side effects you experience and can tell you which side effects might constitute an emergency situation.

- Diuretics (also called "water pills"; see also pages 158–159) help rid the body of excess fluids; this can reduce edema and ease the burden on the heart. Some diuretics deplete the body's potassium reserves. Your doctor will tell you if you need to take supplements or to eat more potassium-rich foods, such as bananas, orange juice, and tomato juice.
- Digitalis medicines help the heart pump with more strength, enabling it to deliver more blood—and therefore higher levels of oxygen—with each beat. Physicians prescribing digitalis for heart-failure patients usually combine it with other drugs such as diuretics and ACE inhibitors.

MEDICINES FOR RELATED CONDITIONS

Controlling other heart problems helps keep heart failure under control, too. Depending on which other heart problems you have, medications may be prescribed to:

- Lower blood pressure (antihypertensives)
- Lower cholesterol levels (statins)
- Prevent blood clots (anticoagulants, such as aspirin)
- Keep the heartbeat steady (antiarrhythmics)

Intravenous (IV) medications. If your heart-failure symptoms become severe, your doctor may recommend that you receive medications through an IV. This approach works quickly to help your heart pump better and relieve your symptoms. You may have to stay in the hospital or another medical facility for a few days until you feel better.

TAKING YOUR MEDICATION

Taking too much medication or too little can hurt your heart. Follow all of your doctor's and pharmacist's instructions. Even if you start to feel better, don't stop taking your medication or change your dosage unless your doctor tells you to.

FOLLOWING A ROUTINE

Having a routine can help you remember when to take your medications. Try these tips:

- Take your pills at the same times each day. If you take them when you routinely do something else, it will help you remember. For instance, take your pills just before you brush your teeth or eat a meal. Ask your doctor or pharmacist which medications can be taken with meals.
- Get a pillbox that's marked with the days of the week; some also feature compartments representing different times of the day. Refill the pillbox at the start of each week. (Most pharmacies sell compartmented pillboxes; see also page 152.)

TRACKING MEDICATIONS

For your medications to work, you must take them exactly as directed. The following tips will help:

- Refill your prescription when you still have a week's supply of pills left so you never run out.
- Keep your medication in your carry-on (not checked) luggage when you travel.
- Maintain an up-to-date list of all the medications you take, including over-the-counter medications and dietary supplements. Show this list to any doctor or dentist who treats you. Also show it to your pharmacist before you buy any prescription or over-the-counter medication. Your pharmacist can tell you which medications might cause problems when taken together.

Medical procedures for heart failure

Certain medical procedures may be able to help you manage heart failure. Typically these procedures address underlying conditions

Be Smart About Alternatives

Claims are being studied that certain herbs and supplements can help with heart-failure symptoms, ut these have yet to be medically proven. Keep in mind that "natural" is not a synonym for "safe"; these products are not approved by the Food and Drug Administration. Some herbs, extracts, and other supplements can interact with prescribed and over-the-counter medications. If you want to try an alternative treatment, talk with your health care provider first. You can also research them yourself at http://ods.od.nih.gov/index.aspx.

affecting your heart, such as artery and valve problems and rhythm irregularities.

PROCEDURES FOR ARTERY AND VALVE PROBLEMS

If you are a heart-failure patient with coronary artery disease or valve disease, certain procedures may improve blood flow and help the heart pump better.

- Angioplasty and stenting expand narrowed coronary arteries; coronary artery bypass surgery reroutes blood around a clogged artery. Pages 177–183 present more detailed information on these procedures.
- Valve surgery repairs or replaces faulty valves so blood can flow properly.

PROCEDURES FOR RHYTHM PROBLEMS

Devices attached to the heart can regulate a slow or abnormal heart rhythm and alleviate heart strain when congestive heart failure is present. See pages 209–212 for more about these devices.

- A pacemaker is a small electronic device that corrects a slow heartbeat. Some pacemakers stimulate only one side of the heart. Others, called biventricular pacemakers, stimulate both sides.
- An implantable cardioverter defibrillator (ICD) treats fast heart rhythms that can become life threatening.

Tracking Your Health

As you deal with heart failure, you'll experience both good and bad days. Staying aware of what's happening in your body may help increase the number of good days. It's especially important to keep tabs on your weight, which should be checked every day. By tracking your symptoms and any drug side effects—and discussing what you've noticed with your health care provider—you can help make your treatment plan more effective.

Weighing yourself

Rapid weight gain can be a sign that you are retaining water and that your treatment plan needs to be changed. To monitor your weight:

- Weigh yourself at the same time on the same scale every morning, wearing the same clothes. Weigh yourself after urinating and before eating.
- Record your weight each day.
- Call your doctor if you gain two or more pounds in one day or if you gain three to five pounds in one week. Your doctor will tell you what to do next.

Your symptom chart

Use a chart to track your weight and heart-failure symptoms. First, copy the blank chart so you'll have a clean one to use each month. Then record your weight each day. Also write down any symptoms you note, such as swelling or shortness of breath. Bring the chart pages with you whenever you visit your health care provider.

Treating Heart-Rhythm Problems

"Arrhythmia" is the term for an abnormal heartbeat. There are several important types of arrhythmia, each requiring separate treatment.

Atrial fibrillation

Atrial fibrillation is a common heart problem that affects 2.5 million Americans. It is caused by misfirings in the heart muscle that make

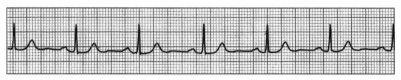

> Normal heart rhythm

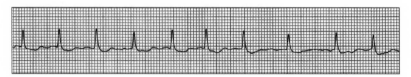

> Atrial fibrillation

the atria (upper chambers of the heart) quiver and pump erratically.

People with atrial fibrillation often experience palpitations (a fast, fluttering heartbeat). They may also have other symptoms such as weakness, shortness of breath, chest pain or tightness, dizziness, and fainting spells. But many people with atrial fibrillation have no symptoms at all.

Atrial fibrillation is a potentially dangerous condition because blood that is not kept on the move can pool and form clots in the atria. These clots can migrate to other parts of the body and cause life-threatening problems, especially strokes.

Atrial fibrillation triggers an estimated 100,000 strokes each year in the U.S.

A painless test called an electrocardiogram (ECG or EKG) is a foolproof way of detecting atrial fibrillation. The test reveals how electrical signals travel through the heart. During an ECG, small pads containing electrodes are placed on your chest, arms, and legs. Wires connect the pads to the ECG machine, which records your heart signals—including any changes that occur during the test. A stress ECG is a specialized test that monitors your heart's electrical activity as you exercise, usually on a treadmill.

An ECG test administered in a doctor's office, clinic, or hospital works well for diagnosing atrial fibrillation in those who have the condition all the time. But in order to pinpoint the intermittent (or "paroxysmal") form of atrial fibrillation, your doctor may have you wear a device called a Holter monitor that measures heart rhythm over an entire day.

For some people whose heart failure is extremely serious and potentially life-threatening, a heart transplant may be an option. In some cases, an artificial pump called a Left Ventricular Assist Device (LVAD) is first attached to the heart to help it pump. The LVAD may serve as a temporary treatment until a healthy heart from a suitable donor becomes available. LVADs can also be kept in place permanently.

Restoring normal rhythm with drugs

Certain antiarrhythmic drugs stop atrial fibrillation and restore normal rhythm, a process called chemical cardioversion. These medications can also help prevent a fast heart rate from starting. Your doctor may prescribe one or more of these drugs; they include amiodarone, flecainide, lidocaine, mexiletine, procainamide, and quinidine.

Drugs that keep clots at bay

Blood clots are a major concern for people with atrial fibrillation. You may be given an anticoagulant to prevent this from happening.

Aspirin is sometimes used as an anticoagulant. Coumadin® (warfarin) is a prescription anticoagulant that requires regular blood tests to ensure that the dose is neither too high nor too low. The test results come in the form of a number called protime or INR. Always know your current protime/INR and when your next blood test is due. Follow through with all required tests and make sure your physician gets the results promptly so your dosage can be adjusted if need be.

Taking warfarin carries some risks, among them excessive bleeding. Pregnant women and women trying to conceive should avoid warfarin because of its risk of birth defects. Certain drugs can affect how warfarin works. Aspirin, for example, can boost the anticoagulant effect of warfarin, increasing the risk of uncontrollable bleeding. If you are taking warfarin, always ask your doctor before taking any other medications, including ones bought without a prescription.

Alcohol can also affect warfarin, so limit wine, beer, and hard liquor to no more than one or two drinks per day. Alcohol not only affects how your body uses warfarin but—combined with the medication's anti-clotting action—can also cause bleeding of the stomach lining.

WATCHING WHAT YOU EAT

The following foods are high in vitamin K, which can offset the effects of warfarin. For warfarin to work as it should, keep the total amount of these foods the same each day:

- Asparagus
- Avocado
- Broccoli
- Brussels sprouts
- Cabbage
- Coleslaw
- Collard greens
- Endive
- Kale
- Lettuce
- Mustard greens
- Sauerkraut
- Soybeans
- Spinach
- Swiss chard
- Turnip greens

HELPFUL HINTS WHEN USING WARFARIN

Because warfarin keeps your blood from clotting, you also need to protect yourself from injury. Follow these tips to protect yourself from excessive bleeding:

- Take warfarin at the same time each day (preferably at night). If you miss a dose, take the next one at the normal time. Never take two doses at once.
- Have blood tests (protime or INR) done as often as directed. This is the only way to check if your dosage is right.

Foods That Affect Warfarin

Vitamin K encourages your blood to clot. That's why eating foods containing vitamin K can counteract the blood-thinning effects of warfarin. You needn't avoid foods containing vitamin K, but you should keep the amount of them you eat steady (the same from day to day). If you change your diet for any reason—because of an illness, for example, or to lose weight—be sure to tell your health care provider.

- Check with your health care provider before taking any other medications.
- Use a soft toothbrush and floss gently to minimize the risk of bleeding.
- Use an electric razor to avoid shaving cuts.
- Don't go barefoot. Don't trim corns or calluses yourself.
- Protect yourself from falling. Wear shoes with nonskid soles. Use nonskid rubber mats on floors. Remove throw rugs. And don't play rough contact sports.
- Tell all your health care providers, including your dentist, that you are on Coumadin®. Wear a medical-alert bracelet.

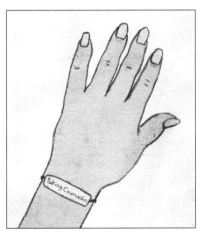

> Wear identification that says you're taking Coumadin®.
  Medical personnel will need to know this if you're injured.

Electrical cardioversion

If chemical cardioversion (the use of antiarrhythmic medications) doesn't successfully treat your arrhythmia, the next step may be electrical cardioversion—a procedure that uses electricity to restore your heart's normal rhythm.

During electrical cardioversion, the doctor gives your heart a brief electric shock that momentarily stops all electrical activity in the heart, including the irregular signals that cause your atrial fibrillation; a regular, normal heart rhythm can then take over. In some people, more than one electric-shock treatment may be necessary to restore a normal rhythm. In others, the procedure may not work at all.

Special pads containing electrodes are placed on your chest and connected to an ECG machine that shows your heartbeat. An IV line supplies a drug that makes you sleepy. You will not feel any discomfort during the procedure. Paddles placed on your chest and back send a very brief electric shock to your heart. Your heartbeat is monitored on the ECG throughout the test.

Catheter ablation

Chemical and electrical cardioversion sometimes don't arrest atrial fibrillation. Even when such cardioversions work, they often are only temporarily effective. A procedure called catheter ablation may provide longer-lasting relief. It destroys a few of the cells in the atria that are causing the fast heart rhythm.

During catheter ablation, a special catheter is inserted through a blood vessel into the heart. The tip of the catheter is positioned at the cells causing the rhythm problem. Energy is then sent through the catheter to ablate, or destroy, some of those cells. Because this energy usually takes the form of radio waves, the procedure is sometimes called radiofrequency catheter ablation.

A study published in the March 2006 issue of the *New England Journal of Medicine* reported that most people with a long history of atrial fibrillation can get long-lasting relief from radiofrequency catheter ablation. In clinical trials, the two-hour procedure restored normal rhythm in 74 percent of patients. A year after the procedure, these patients remained free of their irregular heartbeat.

Treating ventricular fibrillation

Ventricular fibrillation causes the heart's lower chambers—the ventricles—to beat quickly and unevenly. It's a life-threatening arrhythmia because it can lead to cardiac arrest (when the heart quivers instead of pumping), which in turn can cause sudden death. About 400,000 people die each year in the United States as a result of ventricular arrhythmias.

People who have survived a cardiac arrest caused by ventricular fibrillation are at increased risk of a repeat episode. Ventricular tachycardia—a related condition in which the ventricles beat very fast—also raises the risk of cardiac arrest because it can progress to ventricular fibrillation.

Medications can reduce these risks. But another treatment option—an implantable cardioverter defibrillator, or ICD—may pro-

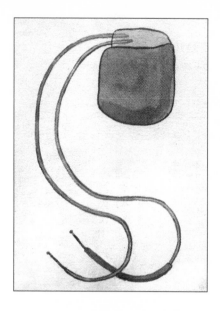

> The ICD generator is a smooth, lightweight metal case containing a tiny computer and a battery. The generator tracks heart rhythm and sends out electrical impulses and shocks as needed. The leads are wires covered by soft, flexible plastic. An ICD may have one or more leads that carry electrical impulses from the generator to the heart.

vide even better protection against episodes of ventricular fibrillation or tachycardia. ICDs have been found to be 99 percent effective in preventing such episodes.

An ICD is a small computerized electronic device that is implanted inside the body. It tracks your heart rhythm and administers small, painless shocks to the heart if it senses that tempo becoming dangerously fast. But if the even deadlier chaotic rhythm of ventricular fibrillation occurs, the ICD takes more drastic action, emitting a potentially life-saving but painful shock. The shock from an ICD will not harm your body—nor can it hurt anyone near you.

An ICD can do one or more of the following:

Antitachycardia pacing (ATP): The ICD can send out a series of signals to compete with and override a fast rhythm. This may feel like a fluttering in your chest—or you may not feel it at all.

Cardioversion: If ATP doesn't slow a fast rhythm, the ICD can give the heart one or more small shocks. These stop the fast rhythm.

Defibrillation: If the ICD senses a very fast, irregular rhythm, it quickly sends a strong shock to the heart. This stops the heart for a second, giving it a chance to revert to its normal rhythm. Defibrillation may feel as strong as a kick in the chest.

Bradycardia pacing: As well as slowing a fast heart rhythm, an ICD can correct a heartbeat that is too slow (bradycardia). This can happen if you have a second heart-rhythm problem that causes a slow heartbeat; your heart may also beat too slowly after an ICD shock.

Biventricular pacing (also called cardiac resynchronization therapy): If you have heart failure, the beating of the two ventricles may be out of sync. Biventricular pacing fixes the timing of the ventricles' beats so blood is pumped more efficiently.

IMPLANTING THE ICD

1. ICD implantation can be done in an operating room, an electrophysiology lab, or a cardiac catheterization lab. It does not require major surgery. The process takes one to four hours.

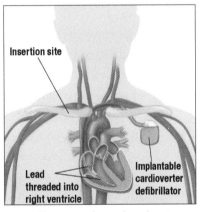

Insertion site

Lead threaded into right ventricle

Implantable cardioverter defibrillator

> An ICD constantly monitors heart rhythm.

   - First, an incision is made in the skin below the collarbone to create a small "pocket" to hold the ICD.
   - A lead is threaded through the incision into a vein in the upper chest. With the help of x-ray monitors, the lead is then guided into one of the heart's chambers.

2. This process may be repeated to guide other leads into other chambers. The leads attach to the heart muscle so they will stay in place.

3. The generator is attached to the leads, and the generator is then placed in its pocket under the skin. The incision is stitched closed.

A 2005 FDA study found that ICDs malfunction nearly five times more frequently than pacemakers. ICD risks include:

- Bleeding or severe bruising
- Puncture of a lung or the heart muscle
- Tearing of the blood-vessel wall
- Clotting or air bubbles in the blood vessel
- Infection or nerve damage at the incision site
- Heart attack, stroke, or death (rare)

Treatment for Heart-Valve Disease

Heart-valve disease occurs when a heart valve—the flaps that let blood move between the chambers of the heart—fails to open or close the way it should. There are four valves in the heart: the tricuspid valve, the pulmonic valve, the mitral valve, and the aortic valve. Any one of these can develop a problem. Your doctor will explain which problem you have and which valve is affected.

Valve disease causes the heart to work harder than normal to move blood. Symptoms include breathing problems, tiredness, chest pain, swollen ankles, and fainting. Over time, heart-valve disease can also tire and weaken the heart muscle. Valve disease can be serious—but it can also be treated.

Problems opening (stenosis)

Sometimes scarring or deposits of calcium may make the valve stiff. When the valve can't open all the way, the problem is called stenosis. Because the blood must now flow through a narrower opening, the heart muscle must work harder to push the blood through.

Problems closing (insufficiency)

Sometimes the flaps of a valve become loose or torn. When a valve can't close all the way, blood can leak backward through the valve, and the heart has to push that blood through the valve again.

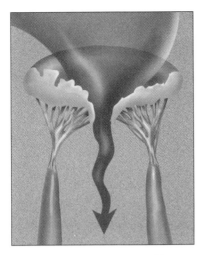

> Stenosis: When a valve is unable to open wide enough, the blood must flow through a smaller opening.

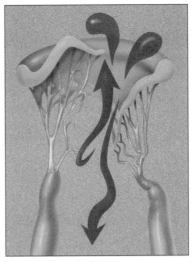

> Insufficiency: When a valve doesn't close tightly, blood leaks backward.

Types of treatment for heart-valve disease

Heart-valve disease often requires no treatment—just regular monitoring to guarantee symptoms aren't getting worse. Based on the type and severity of your valve disease, however, your health care provider may recommend treatment that includes medication or surgery.

MEDICATIONS FOR HEART-VALVE DISEASE

Some medications help ease the symptoms of heart-valve disease; others help prevent problems that valve disease can cause. Remember to inform your provider of every over-the-counter or prescription medication, herb, or supplement you're taking.

MEDICATIONS FOR SYMPTOMS OF VALVE DISEASE

The following medications may be prescribed for the symptoms of valve disease:

Diuretics (pages 158–159) help rid the body of excess fluid, easing the burden on the heart. Getting rid of extra water can also help reduce swelling and shortness of breath.

Digitalis medicines (Digoxin, for example, or Laxonin) help the heart pump with more strength; this enables the heart to pump more blood with each beat. Digitalis medicines may also keep the heartbeat regular.

ACE inhibitors (pages 161–163) relax blood vessels and lower blood pressure. This allows the heart to work less hard to pump the same amount of blood.

Beta blockers (pages 160–161), also used to treat hypertension and angina, slow heart rate, easing the heart's workload.

Antiarrhythmics (pages 205–207)control a fast or irregular heartbeat (palpitations).

OTHER MEDICATIONS FOR HEART-VALVE DISEASE

Problems with heart valves increase the likelihood of clot formation in the heart and also can lead to infection. Medications that help prevent these problems include:

Anticoagulants, which prevent blood clots from forming inside the heart chambers or on a damaged heart valve.

Antibiotics, which help prevent infection due to bacteria that can stick to abnormal heart valves. Your doctor may have you take antibiotics preventively before certain procedures, such as any dental work (including routine cleanings).

Surgery for heart-valve disease

If a malfunctioning heart valve is deemed especially dangerous, it can be surgically repaired or replaced. Repair means that flaws in an existing valve are corrected. Replacement means your own diseased valve is removed and a new valve is put in its place. Your cardiologist or surgeon can tell you more about your surgery, its risks and benefits, and how best to prepare for it.

REPAIRING A VALVE

Certain valve problems can be repaired:

- For insufficiency: Extra tissue is removed or parts of the valve are strengthened to help it close more tightly.
- For stenosis: A catheter is inserted through a blood vessel until it reaches the valve. A balloon on the end of the tube is then inflated inside the valve, stretching the valve open so it can move freely.

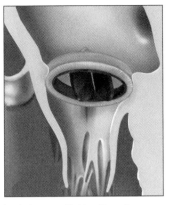

> A ring may tighten the valve opening.

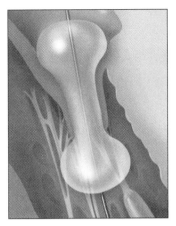

> A balloon may be expanded to open the valve.

REPLACING A VALVE

If the valve can't be repaired, it can be replaced with a prosthetic (substitute) valve. You and your doctor can decide what kind of prosthetic heart valve is best for you.

- Mechanical valves consist of manmade materials. They carry a risk of blood clots forming on their surface, so lifelong therapy with anticoagulant medications is usually required.
- Biological (tissue) valves are taken from pig, cow, or human donors. These valves don't last as long as mechanical valves, but they may not necessitate long-term anticoagulant therapy.

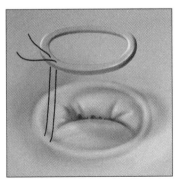

> A replacement valve is positioned in the valve opening and sewn into place.

Recovering Physically & Emotionally 7

You may have recently suffered a heart attack or been diagnosed with heart disease and undergone a procedure, such as balloon angioplasty or bypass surgery, designed to stave off a heart attack. In either case, you need to recover in two ways: physically, with a cardiac-rehabilitation program designed to help you maintain a healthier heart, and emotionally, by learning to deal with the stress, depression, and other problems (including sexual dysfunction) that a heart attack or a diagnosis of heart disease can bring about. This chapter describes the process of rebounding both physically and emotionally from heart disease.

Acceptance Can Lead to Progress

After heart problems or surgery, you may feel depressed and angry. You may have trouble accepting that you're ill. But just as denial is a common response to any serious diagnosis, acceptance is the difficult first step on the road to getting better.

Try to understand that unless you make some changes in your life, you are at high risk for more problems. Think about the rewards of improving your heart health. Once you accept that you must take action to improve your health, you may find it easier to change your lifestyle. If you discover you are struggling, remember that you need not go it alone: Having your family and friends support you and work with you can ease the process of change.

> More than 100,000 people participate in cardiac-rehabilitation and secondary-prevention programs every year.

Also keep in mind that recovery takes time. You will have some good days and some bad days, but gradually you should begin feeling better. Focus on goals that are important to you: returning to work, becoming active again, spending more time with your family. Record your progress on a calendar or in a journal.

Cardiac Rehab & Secondary Prevention: A Second Chance for Your Heart

Until the middle of the last century, heart-attack survivors were thought to have reached the end of their productive lives. Survivors were told they'd have to "take it easy from now on." Treatment typically consisted of several weeks of bed rest—which often left them feeling very weak.

It was a vicious cycle. The enforced rest deconditioned the heart-attack patients' bodies and made them feel exhausted, but they interpreted the exhaustion as a heart-attack complication—which made them even more fearful about becoming active again. All too often, such people were left feeling constantly worried about having another heart attack and thus afraid to go back to work or resume previous activities.

Over the past few decades, by contrast, doctors and patients have come to realize that a heart attack need not put an end to active living. Today, it is widely accepted that the great majority of heart-attack survivors—as well as people who have undergone angioplasty or bypass surgery—can pick up essentially where they left off: They can return to work and resume normal activities—including an active sex life.

A heart attack is a life-threatening event, to be sure, and bypass surgery or angioplasty can be just as traumatic. But any of these experiences can also mark a new beginning—a turning point toward a healthier way of living. Indeed, many heart-attack patients end up feeling healthier than they had for several years leading up to their attack.

Much of the credit goes to cardiac-rehabilitation programs, which have become key to both physical and emotional recovery.

Cardiac rehab is a total program for heart health. Usually designed by a team of rehab specialists, ideally it is tailored to the individual needs of the patient.

Who Needs Cardiac Rehab?

Cardiac-rehabilitation programs initially focused on people who had suffered heart attacks. Nowadays doctors recognize that rehabilitation is just as important for people who have undergone heart-disease procedures such as bypass surgery or angioplasty, or those who have stable coronary artery disease—that is, heart disease that has stabilized over time but might worsen without rehab.

A Team Effort

During cardiac rehab, you will learn how to reduce your risk of future problems. Your doctor can tell you when you are ready to start a rehab program; treatment may even get under way while you're still in the hospital. Programs are available on an inpatient or outpatient basis and in other, non-hospital settings.

The diverse group of professionals making up a cardiac-rehab team brings together all the expertise required to evaluate your heart condition and develop a suitable rehabilitation plan. Team members also serve you by answering your questions about medications, diet, exercise, and—especially during the early stages of cardiac rehab—suitable levels of sexual activity.

Your primary care physician or cardiologist may be part of a team that includes nursing staff, physical therapist, psychologist, cardiac-rehab coordinator, exercise physiologist, social worker, nutritionist, and—if appropriate—smoking-cessation counselor. You will also undoubtedly spend time with other rehab patients who understand what you're going through and with whom you can share your feelings.

Battling Risk Factors

One of the major goals of any cardiac-rehab program is to help you control the risk factors—smoking, inactivity, stress, high blood pressure, and diabetes, among others—that contribute to heart disease. Dealing with risk factors is more than a mere preventive measure; it can also stop an existing case of heart disease from getting worse, thereby reducing the chance of another heart attack.

What's more, the risk factors that cause coronary arteries to become diseased can also affect arteries elsewhere in the body (including the brain, where blockages can lead to a stroke or other serious problems). So reducing your risk of coronary artery disease (CAD) likewise reduces your risk of stroke. This is known as secondary prevention.

Assess your risk factors by answering the questions below. The more times you answer "Yes," the more important it is to change your lifestyle to prevent further harm and aid your recovery.

	YES	NO
• Smoking: Do you smoke cigarettes or use tobacco?	____	____
• Inactivity: Do you avoid exercise or physical activity?	____	____
• High blood cholesterol: Do you eat lots of high-cholesterol foods (such as egg yolks and red meat)? Do you eat lots of saturated fat (such as fried foods and high-fat dairy products)?	____	____
• Obesity: Has your doctor told you that you are overweight?	____	____
• Stress: Do you often feel angry and overstressed?	____	____
• Related conditions: Do you have high blood blood pressure (hypertension) or diabetes?	____	____
• Family history: Is there a history of heart disease, early heart attacks, or diabetes in your family?	____	____

You can't change your family history, obviously, but you can control many of the other risk factors associated with heart disease. Stopping smoking, eating a healthy diet, learning to handle stress, and getting regular exercise can and should become key elements in your rehab program. (See Chapter 3 for more about risk factors and how to control them.) Keep in mind that risk factors are additive: The greater number of risk factors you have, the higher the risks.

Addressing even a single risk factor can require a major lifestyle change—especially if the target behavior has become ingrained in your everyday life. If you are naturally a hard-driving person, you may need to work hard at relaxing more (as ironic as that sounds) and make downtime a part of your regular schedule. If you've always been overweight, you will need to find a way to lose those extra pounds and keep them off. If you've smoked for years and tried to quit unsuccessfully, now is the time to put all your effort into stopping for good. Changing such deeply entrenched habits is never easy, but you have about the best motivation going: Your health—perhaps even your life—depends on it.

> Many patients report that learning to handle stress more effectively was the most important change they made after their cardiac event.

The Exercise Angle

The other cornerstone of a cardiac-rehab program is exercise. Regular exercise improves the condition of your heart and coronary arteries. It also lowers blood pressure, relieves stress, and can help you control your weight.

Your doctor and other members of the cardiac-rehab team will design an exercise program tailored to your needs and your current condition. They will ensure that you engage in the right level of exercise at the right time. Yes, you can do too much too soon, but bear in mind that your heart is a muscle—and that exercise will make it stronger and help it function more efficiently.

A supervised exercise program

Your cardiac-rehab exercise program may begin right in the hospital under the supervision of your doctor or cardiologist. Your first goal will be to regain basic strength, and your first exercises will be relatively light—perhaps as simple as walking up and down the hallway outside your room. After you leave the hospital, you may continue supervised exercise at a medical center or other facility. Alternatively, you may be directed to follow a program at home. These more advanced exercises will help you build strength, flexibility, and endurance.

Facing the challenge

If you've never exercised before, the prospect of unfamiliar workout routines and sweating it up at the gym may leave you cold. But it need not be that way at all. You can jump-start your new, healthier existence simply by focusing on ways to become more active in your day-to-day life. Small changes in how you do things throughout the day can add up to a significant improvement in your activity level.

Most cardiac-rehab programs aim to get you active for 30 minutes a day most days of the week—and ideally every day. But that should be your ultimate goal, not what you need to accomplish right away. The key is to start slowly and acclimate yourself to being more active. You can add other forms of exercise and expend more energy as you feel able.

Evaluating your exercise tolerance

Before you start an exercise program, your cardiac-rehab team will assess your current state of health, which may involve a stress test to see how your heart responds to exercise (see pages 77–79). The results of this and other evaluations will help determine what sort of exercise program is right for you.

Virtually everyone who has had a heart attack can benefit from cardiac rehab.

It's natural to worry that too much activity might cause chest pain or bring on a heart attack (you may be particularly concerned if you've already experienced such a trauma). But, with proper evaluation, your team can tailor an exercise plan that allows you to start slowly and progress safely.

Types of exercise for cardiac rehab

Aerobic exercise improves the functioning of your heart, lungs, and blood vessels. You breathe harder, your heart beats faster, and you might sweat a bit. Examples of aerobic exercise are walking or jogging, cycling, and swimming.

Exercise vs. Angioplasty

In March 2004, the American Heart Association journal *Circulation* published the results of a study comparing angioplasty and increased exercise as treatments for heart disease. The study divided 101 older men with stable (not worsening over time) CAD into two groups: One group underwent angioplasty; men in the other group followed a one-year exercise program of pedaling a stationary bicycle 20 minutes every day.

By the end of the year, 30 percent of the angioplasty group had experienced a heart attack or other coronary event, whereas only 12 percent of the exercisers had. The authors concluded that angioplasty can improve the health of the majority of patients with stable CAD, but that it should be combined with a more aggressive lifestyle intervention, including daily physical exercise.

Strength exercises build muscles. When your muscles are stronger, your heart rate becomes less elevated when you exert yourself and your blood pressure stays under control. Strength exercises typically involve lifting weights or doing situps, pushups, or other routines that target specific muscles (or muscle groups).

Stretching after exercise helps prevent injury. Stretching also keeps your muscles relaxed and reduces stress.

Heart help from aerobic exercise

Aerobic exercise helps your heart and other muscles use oxygen more efficiently. Many cardiac-rehab programs use walking on a treadmill as a basic form of aerobic exercise. Some programs also use other equipment such as stationary bikes, arm cranks, or light weights. At least at the beginning and perhaps on a continuing basis, your heart rate and blood pressure will be monitored while you exercise.

SETTING THE PACE

The talk test is an easy way to set a good pace for yourself. Try talking as you exercise. If you can talk and carry on a conversation, you're exercising at about the right level of exertion. If you're too out of breath to talk comfortably, slow down a bit. If you can sing without trouble, exercise a little harder. Find a pace that lets you talk for more than a few minutes at a time.

A more refined form of pace-setting gauges exertion by your heart rate. Discuss with your doctor whether you should be aiming for a "target zone" heart rate during aerobic exercise. Target zones are ranges of heartbeats per minute (such as 100 to 140 bpm or 80 to 120 bpm) that represent the level at which exercise increases the oxygen demands on your heart enough to give it a good workout but not so much as to overstress it. For people in good health, age determines the appropriate target zone: The older you are, the lower your target zone. Your doctor's analysis of the condition of your heart will help determine what your target zone should be.

TAKING YOUR PULSE

Taking your pulse is one way to measure your heart rate to see if you are meeting your target-zone heart rate. The pulsing you feel in your wrist represents the pace at which your heart is beating as it pumps blood through your body. The heart responds to the increased demands of exercise by beating faster to supply the body with more oxygen-bearing blood. To determine if you're below, above, or within your target zone, you may be asked to take your pulse regularly during or after exercise or when you feel something is wrong. Here's how to do it:

Find Your Pulse

- With your first two fingers, press lightly on the inside of your wrist, just below the base of the thumb. You should not be pressing on a bone or on any of the tendons in your wrist.
- Feel for a steady pulsing and continue pressing just firmly enough to detect the beat. If you have trouble finding your pulse, move your fingers slightly to a new spot, or try your other wrist.

Take Your Pulse

- Count the number of beats you feel in your wrist in a given amount of time. Heart rate is always expressed as beats per minute (bpm), but you don't necessarily have to count for a full minute. Most people count for six seconds and then multiply by 10 to equal a minute or count for 10 seconds and then multiply by six.

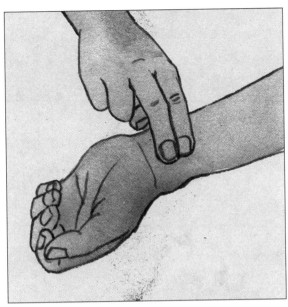

> To take your pulse, press until you feel light beating.

- Check with your doctor about timing your pulse. If you're supposed to gauge how quickly your heart returns to a resting rate after exercise, for example, you'll want to count for only 6 or 10 seconds to get quick snapshots of your pulse at different times.
- A normal "resting" pulse is 60 to 100 beats per minute; the beats should be regular and evenly spaced. Talk to your doctor about your own targets and anything particular to your condition you should be watching for.

Record the Results

Write down your pulse every time you take it or as your doctor advises. You can use the chart on page 226 or make one of your own. Be prepared to take your results with you whenever you visit the doctor.

ANOTHER WAY TO GAUGE EXERTION

In addition to checking your pulse, you can measure exertion by using the Borg RPE Scale, which gauges how hard you are working by what the exercise feels like. This chart appears on page 227.

Signs of Overexertion

Stop exercising and call your doctor if you feel any of these symptoms:

- Chest pain or discomfort
- Burning, tightness, heaviness, or pressure in your chest
- Unusual aching in your arm, shoulder, neck, jaw, or back
- Trouble catching your breath
- Racing or skipping heartbeat
- Extreme fatigue (especially after exercise)
- Lightheadedness, dizziness, or nausea

Date	Time	Beats per Minute	Is It Regular?	Activity Just Before Taking Pulse
			Yes No	
			Yes No	
			Yes No	
			Yes No	
			Yes No	
			Yes No	
			Yes No	
			Yes No	
			Yes No	
			Yes No	
			Yes No	
			Yes No	

The Borg RPE Scale lets you rate your exertion by how hard the exercise feels to you. As you exercise, take note of how hard your muscles are working and how breathless you are. Then look at the scale below and rate your response as objectively as possible.

Level	How It Feels	Level	How It Feels	Level	How It Feels
6	No exertion at all	11	Light	17	Very hard
7	Extremely light	12		18	
8		13	Somewhat hard	19	Extremely hard
9	Very light	14		20	Maximum exertion
10		15	Hard (heavy)		
		16			

Scale © 1985 by Gunnar Borg

CONTINUING AT HOME

Some people stay in supervised exercise programs at a medical center or gym; others transition into continuing on their own, either at a fitness center or at home. The most important thing is to stick with it. By continuing with a program of exercise, you lower your risk for a heart attack or stroke in the future. (You'll feel and look better, too.) The more you make exercise a part of your life, the greater benefit you're likely to get from being active.

A common pitfall for people who start exercising on their own is that they set their sights too high. Remember, the goal is not to become an Olympic athlete. Talk to your doctor about devising an exercise plan you will enjoy. It should fit your budget and schedule and feature reasonable, achievable goals. Meeting targets is one of the best ways to stay motivated.

What constitutes an enjoyable exercise? That truly is up to you. Some people prefer familiar activities; others like to challenge themselves with something new, or continually shift among several choices for variety. Check off any of the following activities that fit the bill for you, or write in others:

Walking

Jogging

Swimming

Cycling

Aerobics class

Ballroom dancing

Golf

Hiking

Stair climbing

Roller skating or in-line skating

Water sports or water exercises

CHEER, NOT CHORE

When it comes to fabricating excuses not to exercise, everyone—heart patient or no—seems capable of endless invention. Indeed, look on exercise as a chore and those excuses become a snap to create. The best way *not* to dodge exercise, therefore, is to make the undertaking as enjoyable as you can. Try the tips below to boost your enjoyment—and to overcome the obstacles that typically crop up.

- Not enough time to exercise? Try a few minutes of gardening before dinner or a 10-minute walk at lunch. You need not achieve your goal of 30 minutes of daily exercise in a single uninterrupted workout. It's okay to accumulate that 30-minute total here and there in the course of a day.
- Try exercising at different times during the day to see what's best for you—and which time you enjoy the most.
- Easily bored working out by yourself? Cardiac-rehab classes may have shown you that exercising with a group can keep you motivated. Join a walking club or an exercise group at your local health club or YMCA, or try exercising with a friend.
- Put off by the expense of a gym or fancy home equipment? All you need for an effective exercise program are a pair of sturdy sneakers or running shoes and a place to walk; you can do strength exercises with simple handheld weights.

TIPS FOR PEOPLE WITH DIABETES

Exercise is vitally important if you have diabetes. It can help control both diabetes itself and the heart disease often associated with diabetes. Follow these tips:

- Check to make sure that your blood sugar is within a safe range before exercise. If you're unsure about your safe range, ask your doctor.

- Eat a snack an hour or two before you exercise.
- Drink a full glass of water before and after any major activity.
- Carry glucose tablets or hard candy to raise your blood-sugar level in a hurry if you need to.
- Check your feet for sores or blisters before and after you exercise.

For other questions about diabetes and exercise, check with your health care provider.

Recovering Emotionally from Heart Disease

Having a heart attack or undergoing a heart-disease procedure such as bypass surgery or angioplasty is not just physically traumatic. For many people, such events leave a major emotional impact as well.

Within days of the event, many people find themselves feeling depressed, often because they fear a loss of physical ability. This depression can be mild and brief, or it can be severe and long-lasting.

Are You Depressed?

Feeling sad or overwhelmed at times is a normal part of life. But if sad feelings persist for more than a few days, you may be clinically depressed. You should inform your doctor if you do any of the following:

- Lose interest in food, sex, or other things that you previously enjoyed.
- Sleep much less or much more.
- Have thoughts of suicide.
- Feel hopeless about the future.
- Cry more than usual.
- Can't get through your normal routine.
- Cannot concentrate.
- React irritably much of the time.

Most cardiac-rehab programs, recognizing that depression is a common outgrowth of heart attack or procedures for treating heart disease, start helping patients and their families address the problem as soon as possible. Never hesitate to report that you're feeling depressed; it's nothing to be ashamed of, and the sooner you seek help the faster you will feel better.

Sex, Intimacy & Heart Disease

People who have had heart trouble often develop strong negative emotions that interfere with more tender feelings of intimacy and sexual desire. You may find that you are fearful about the future or anxious about your ability to enjoy sex. Anger that this has happened to you may overwhelm virtually every other emotion. But as your body heals, sexual desire is likely to return. When you and your partner are ready, there's no reason you can't renew your sexual relationship.

Your feelings are normal

Even when you feel ready to resume sexual activity, you're likely to have concerns and troubling emotions. At first you may be afraid that any activity, including sex, could cause pain or injury. Your partner may share these fears. Worrying about your physical appearance is common as well. Bear in mind that these feelings are normal and that it's good to be open about them. Discuss these issues with your partner. The key is to tell each other about your needs—emotional as well as sexual.

Rebuilding intimacy

An intimate relationship is built on shared feelings. The stress and anxiety of a heart attack or surgery can hinder open communication, possibly even triggering sexual problems that were not present before. Talking honestly with your partner is the first step toward rebuilding intimacy.

Don't hesitate to remind one another that misgivings about sex in these situations are normal. Your own concerns will most likely subside as you begin to feel better. Keep the communication going as you work through any feelings of fear, depression, anger, or sadness.

When you both feel ready for sex, start slowly. Relax and enjoy each other. Above all, try not to worry. Remember that having sex takes only about as much energy as climbing two short flights of stairs.

Intimacy after heart surgery

If you've had heart surgery, ask your doctor when you can resume sex. Once you're given the okay, be reassured that your incisions will not rupture—nor will you otherwise damage your heart—during sex. While you're healing, you may want to try the following to prevent pain during sex:

- Try positions that put less strain on your chest. Experiment until you find what works best for you.
- Avoid twisting motions until your sternum (breastbone) has had a chance to fully heal.

Taking the first step

Knowing what's troubling you is the first step toward overcoming negative feelings. Start with these positive action steps:

- Acknowledge what you feel.
- Be patient with yourself.
- Talk with your partner about your feelings.

Remember, there is no need to prove yourself. But when you feel ready for sex, it's safe to go ahead.

Talking with your partner

Some people find it difficult to discuss their feelings, yet bottling them up will only make you and your partner feel you're in this thing alone. Talking openly, by contrast, can help you understand and resolve any conflicted emotions. It can also help reduce stress. When you talk:

- Choose a time when you are both relaxed. Pick a place where you feel at ease and will not be interrupted.

- Listen to each other. Acknowledge one another's concerns and make a sincere effort to understand. Do your best to listen until your partner has finished talking.
- Support each other. Be patient and try not to criticize.

Go slowly

If both partners are not ready for sex, don't force the issue. You can move toward having sex by expressing your love in other ways.

- At first, try hugging, kissing, touching, or caressing. This can help you both feel close and wanted.
- When you feel ready for sex, focus on giving each other pleasure. Foreplay and mutual stimulation can be as important as orgasm.

Some helpful hints

- Choose a time when you both feel rested. This could be when you wake up in the morning or after you have taken a nap.
- Wait at least an hour after eating, taking a bath or shower, or exercising.
- For safety's sake, check with your health care provider before using any erectile dysfunction drugs. Certain types of erectile dysfunction drugs (such as Viagra®, Levitra®, and Cialis®) are dangerous for people who are also taking nitroglycerin products. Ask your health care provider what other options may be available.
- If you suspect that a heart medication is eroding your sexual desire, check with your doctor, who may be able to change the medication or prescribe something to enhance sexual function.
- Try to exercise five days a week. Exercise gives you more energy and helps defuse stress.

If you encounter problems

- When you're dealing with a medical problem such as heart disease, it's not unusual to have trouble becoming aroused.

Talk to your doctor about erectile dysfunction—fairly common in men with heart disease. In most cases, your doctor can prescribe medication to improve sexual function. For women, products such as estrogen cream and lubrication can make sex feel more comfortable.

- If you have angina (chest pain) during sex, stop and take nitroglycerin as prescribed by your doctor. If the angina goes away, you can resume sex.
- If you have shortness of breath during sex, stop for a few minutes. If it doesn't go away, or if it comes back when you resume sex, call your doctor.

For better communication

To help you listen to each other's feelings, try this "talker-listener" approach, a standard technique in professional counseling. One person starts as the "talker," the other as the "listener." The two then switch roles.

1. As the talker, tell your partner up to three things you are feeling. Start each statement with "I" and keep it brief. You might say something like, "I'm afraid that if we make love, I'll get tired and have to stop."
2. Your partner listens but does not say anything until you are through speaking.
3. Next, your partner tells you in his or her own words what you said. You simply listen.
4. Now change roles: Your partner becomes the talker, and you listen. Finally, you tell your partner in your own words what you heard.

Run through the steps as many times as you like in each session. Try this helpful exchange at least three times a week.

When to get help

As you resume your sex life, you may find that certain issues still stand in the way. Strong emotions may make it tough to be candid with your partner. Medications or depression could be affecting

Shun the Blame Game

It's crucial to be open about your emotional reactions, but it's also just as important not to blame your partner for something you may be feeling. This is a difficult time for both of you—a time when most issues have nothing to do with being anyone's fault.

- Remember that negative feelings—both your own and those of your partner—do pass.
- Know that having sex when you're both ready won't harm your partner.
- Be patient. You're both going through a rough period in your lives together. Give yourself time to rebuild intimacy.

your desire or performance. If you're facing these or other problems, don't delay in asking for help.

- Try talking together with your partner to a doctor, nurse, member of the clergy, or counselor. Most cardiac-rehab programs offer sexual counseling.
- If you feel depressed or lack sexual drive, talk to your doctor. Your medications may be affecting your desire or ability to have sex, in which case your doctor may be able to help. You might also be clinically depressed as a result of your heart problem, meaning you may benefit from one-on-one counseling with a therapist or from taking an antidepressant medication.

Treatment Advances on the Horizon 8

WITH HEART DISEASE THE LEADING KILLER of both men and women in the United States, the condition has become the focal point for medical researchers striving to prevent and treat it. This chapter describes some of the most promising results of their research. It discusses advances that are already available, those that may be approved in a few months or years, and therapies still in development that could one day revolutionize the treatment of heart disease. The chapter concludes with a discussion of some new findings about one of the oldest—and most important—heart-disease therapies of all: aspirin.

New Angina Treatment

Each year, nearly seven million Americans are diagnosed with angina—the heart pain that occurs when atherosclerosis narrows coronary arteries, depriving the heart muscle of the oxygen-rich blood it needs. In 2006, the U.S. Food and Drug Administration (FDA) approved the drug ranolazine (Ranexa®) for treating chronic angina.

Ranolazine is the first new drug for relieving angina that has been approved in more than a decade. It was studied in two large clinical trials that involved patients with chronic angina who still had symptoms despite being treated with other anti-angina drugs. The studies showed that although ranolazine cannot eliminate angina, it can reduce the number of weekly angina attacks. In both studies, ranolazine appeared to be less effective for women than for men.

Other types of angina drugs—notably beta blockers, nitrates, and calcium-channel blockers—work by slowing down the heart so it needs less oxygen or by dilating clogged coronary arteries so they deliver more blood to heart muscle. Ranolazine, by contrast, appears to relieve angina in a radically different way: It "persuades" heart-muscle cells to choose sugar, not fat, as their source of energy. Burning sugar for energy requires less oxygen than burning fat, so the heart muscle needs less oxygen—a significant benefit for parts of the heart that are already getting less than their fair oxygen share.

The FDA has ruled that Ranexa be restricted to those patients whose angina cannot be treated by older anti-angina drugs.

Heart-Valve Improvements

According to the American Heart Association, every year more than 78,000 people undergo surgery to replace heart valves. Replacing a heart valve is a grueling procedure: Surgeons saw the sternum (breast bone) in half, then stop the heart, excise the defective valve, and sew in a new one. A week's hospital stay is typically required, followed by two to three months to recover fully. Thousands of patients—those considered too ill or too frail to survive the operation—get turned down for new valves each year.

Fortunately, promising new "closed-heart surgery" techniques may soon allow patients to receive replacement valves with much less surgical trauma. In a pioneering clinical trial, a valve was threaded through a leg artery and up to the heart in much the same way that balloon-angioplasty procedures are now routinely carried out. As of April 2006, nineteen Americans and 80 others worldwide had received replacement heart valves in this fashion. Fourteen people in Germany, Canada, and Austria had received a replacement valve via a more direct route to the heart: through an incision made between two ribs.

Doctors performing these minimally invasive valve replacements don't remove the diseased valve; instead, they prop the old one open and wedge the new valve inside it. Typically, patients can leave the hospital the next day and recover fully from the procedure in less than a month. Three years later, some of the earliest recipients of valves implanted in this way are alive and thriving. "Most of us think this is the future," says Northwestern University heart-valve specialist Robert Bonow, M.D.

Home-Grown Heart Valves

Currently, patients who need a replacement heart valve can choose a mechanical device that will probably last more than 30 years. Alternatively, they can opt for a biological valve (usually a specially treated valve from a pig) that may wear out in 10 years.

Regrettably, both mechanical and biological heart valves are susceptible to infection. And, unlike your "originally issued" heart valves, neither type grows with the patient. Children who need valve replacement must therefore undergo multiple surgical procedures as they age.

An even better choice—and one that may be available in a few years—is a heart valve grown from the patient's own cells. At medical institutions around the world (including Massachusetts General Hospital and the Yale University School of Medicine), researchers known as tissue engineers are working to develop just such a "supervalve"—one that would neither wear out nor require anticoagulants, while at the same time better resisting infections and growing along with the individual.

At Massachusetts General Hospital, a collaborative research project between the Division of Cardiac Surgery and the Tissue Engineering and Organ Fabrication Laboratory led to the development of a tissue-engineered mitral valve that is being evaluated in animals. If these preclinical studies show the valve to be effective, it will be tested in people.

Success in Stopping Failure

People who survive a heart attack may be left with permanent damage to the heart muscle. As a result, their hearts may have a reduced ability to pump blood—a chronic condition known as heart failure. Heart failure hospitalizes one million Americans each year, making it the leading cause of hospital admissions in Medicare recipients. Within 90 days, moreover, 30 percent of patients with heart failure are readmitted to the hospital.

Some evidence suggests that home-based management programs and monitoring can lower these readmission rates—as well as shorten hospital stays for heart-failure patients. Indeed, home-care monitoring can play a key role in providing cost-effective, high-quality care. Simply by reporting their weights and describing any symptoms on a secure website, patients can be monitored by physicians on duty at a remote location. And devices now being investigated can even gauge blood pressure inside the heart and send those readings wirelessly to a website, where a doctor can easily access the information.

Absorbable Stents

In about one-third of cases where balloon angioplasty is used to widen coronary arteries, the widened region of the artery becomes blocked again within six months—a problem known as restenosis, or renarrowing. To prevent restenosis following angioplasty, physicians commonly insert small metal scaffolds, called stents, inside the artery.

German researchers have developed an absorbable stent. A month or so after such a device has propped open an artery, the stent—made almost entirely of easily dissoluble magnesium—is absorbed by the artery's inner wall and disappears. In adults, dissolving stents allow a treated section of a coronary artery to expand and contract in a more natural way. Absorbable stents may be especially useful for children, whose arteries get bigger as they grow up.

Novel Strategies for Raising HDL

Statins, the leading class of cholesterol drugs, do a good job of lowering blood levels of LDL ("bad" cholesterol). But they are only modestly effective at raising levels of HDL, the "good" cholesterol that protects against heart disease by mopping up harmful LDL and transporting it to the liver for disposal. Two drugs that promise to powerfully boost HDL levels may soon be available, however. Each one is described below.

The Milano protein

In the 1980s, researchers found why certain people in the Italian town of Limone sul Garda live such long and healthy lives: They possessed a mutant gene that manufactured an unusual protein, dubbed apo A-1 Milano. This protein armed residents of the town with a highly potent form of HDL, which in turn kept their arteries from clogging.

A company named Esperion Therapeutics has inserted the mutant gene into bacteria that synthesize the Milano protein. The company extracts the protein, purifies it, then places it in artificial HDL particles. With the goal of halting or possibly even reversing coronary-artery clogging, the HDL particles can then be injected into the veins of patients with heart disease.

In 2003, researchers at the Cleveland Clinic reported on a study of 57 heart patients. Some of the patients received injections of this enhanced HDL; others got simple saline injections. After one month, the volume of arterial plaque in patients receiving the Milano protein shrank by an average of 4 percent compared with the patients who had received only the saline placebo.

Meanwhile, the National Institutes of Health is sponsoring a five-year gene-therapy study in which researchers are inserting the Milano gene into animals in a bid to stimulate their tissues to produce a constant supply of the Milano protein.

New Help for Smokers

When tobacco smokers inhale, nicotine reaches the brain within seconds. There it binds to nicotine-receptor molecules on brain cells, activating a "reward pathway" in the brain's circuitry that creates a powerful sense of satisfaction. Gum, patches, and many other products designed to help people stop smoking are mostly controlled-delivery devices; they ease the body's craving for this highly addictive chemical. The smoking-cessation drug known as varenicline tartrate (Champix®) takes a different approach. It latches onto the nicotine receptors and activates them in much the same way that nicotine does, reducing the severity of the smoker's craving for cigarettes as well as the withdrawal symptoms from nicotine. Champix® was being considered for FDA approval in 2006.

Three anti-nicotine vaccines are also in the early stages of development. When someone smokes, the vaccine stimulates the body to produce antibodies that bind to the nicotine entering the bloodstream. This forms a nicotine-antibody complex that is too large to cross from the blood into the brain. With the nicotine unable to reach the brain's nicotine receptors, it cannot activate them. As a result, the smoker obtains none of smoking's customary gratification, making it easier to break the habit. FDA approval of anti-nicotine vaccines is still several years away.

What's Ahead in Weight-Loss Drugs

Only two weight-loss drugs, sibutramine (Meridia®) and orlistat (Xenical®), are currently available. Both cause potentially serious side effects, however, that have discouraged their use.

Several experimental drugs with the potential for fewer side effects are in development. Likeliest to reach the market first is rimonabant (Acomplia®), which could receive FDA approval by 2008. Other weight-loss drugs are being devised as well.

Hypertension & Its Newfound Nemeses

Gene Therapy

Nearly one-third of American adults have high blood pressure (hypertension), a major cause of heart attacks, strokes, and kidney failure. In 2006, University of Florida researchers reported that they had come up with a technique for treating hypertension in the long term. Their goal was to block a protein, called a mineralocorticoid receptor, that signals the bloodstream to absorb sodium and water. This influx boosts the volume of blood in the body—which, naturally enough, raises blood pressure.

The Florida researchers used a technique called RNA interference to block the receptor protein in rats. First, a harmless virus ferried fragments of RNA—the molecular cousin of DNA—into the rats' bodies. These fragments then penetrated individual cells, where they stopped production of the protein by interfering with the gene that coded for it.

Although this experimental treatment kept blood pressure from rising in the rats, it did not lower it to normal levels—perhaps, the researchers surmise, because the animals were monitored for only three weeks after treatment. (In a rare laboratory lagniappe, the researchers discovered that blocking the protein dramatically reduced kidney damage in the rats as well.)

"This new technique can efficiently inhibit the protein and prevent the progression of hypertension," said Dr. Zhongjie Sun, an assistant professor at the University of Florida and the lead author of a study summarizing the group's work. "I'm optimistic that [the method] will be used for human gene therapy to treat hypertension."

Not Your Grandfather's Hypertension

The first in a new class of antihypertension drugs may be available within a few years in the United States. That's notable because aliskiren (Rasilez®) would be the first new hypertension therapy to appear since 1994.

Aliskiren belongs to a class of antihypertensive drugs called renin inhibitors. Renin, an enzyme produced in the kidneys, regulates blood pressure when it is released into the bloodstream. But renin is a "one-way" agent only; it makes blood vessels constrict, boosting your blood pressure. Aliskiren works to lower that pressure by reducing renin levels in the blood,.

Studies have shown Aliskiren to be effective as a single treatment for patients with mild to moderate hypertension. Patients appear to tolerate the drug well, and a large majority—more than 95 percent, in one study—stick with the treatment. One reason for the compliance: The drug can be taken by mouth just once a day.

Bowling Alone

Researchers at Seoul National University in South Korea have developed a way to measure blood pressure using a special apparatus fitted beneath a toilet seat, reported a 2006 issue of *Physiological Measurement*.

The toilet-seat blood-pressure monitor is deemed to be nonintrusive and convenient for everyday use in the home. These traits make it particularly useful for long-term blood-pressure monitoring.

The device calculates blood pressure via contact between the subject's thigh skin and three copper-coated electrodes placed on the toilet seat. Two technologies are used. One is photoplethysmography—a noninvasive technique that measures the volume of blood sent through a patch of tissue with each heartbeat. The second technique is electrocardiography, in which the activity of the heart is recorded electronically.

In a small study, blood pressures calculated when subjects were on the toilet seat were quite similar to their blood pressures measured the standard way. Now prepare to be bowled over: Further refinements may enable blood-pressure results to be transmitted wirelessly from the toilet seat directly to the physician's office.

Patches for Damaged Hearts

After a heart attack, the heart may develop large areas of nonfunctioning scar tissue. Occasionally, a heart transplant is the only solution for the heart failure that can result from this. Yet the demand for donor organs far exceeds the supply.

One promising alternative is to make new heart tissue in the laboratory. Such a "cardiac patch" is a living, beating piece of heart tissue. The patch is grown over several days inside a special chamber called a bioreactor, which replicates the natural growing conditions of heart cells. The cardiac patch is then stitched into a heart that has been damaged by heart attack or chronic disease.

Just as in the developing heart, the artificially grown cells must be densely packed together; they must also be well oxygenated. Not only that, but artificial electrical stimulation is required to mimic the electrical impulses that keep the human heart beating.

Biomedical engineers from Columbia University Medical Center in New York City reported on their successful efforts to grow cardiac patches in 2006. They showed a video of postage-stamp-size cardiac patches beating in the same rhythm as real heart tissue. Several years may elapse, however, before heart patches find their way into actual human hearts.

Let's Build a Better Blood Vessel

Some people—particularly older patients with heart disease—need to have blockages in their coronary arteries bypassed, but they lack suitable vessels of their own to serve as replacements. According to a 2005 study published in the medical journal *The Lancet,* Duke University researchers have demonstrated that new human blood vessels can be grown from cells taken from the very patients they are intended to benefit.

The Duke researchers removed cells from the saphenous veins of four men, ages 47 to 74, who happened to be undergoing coronary artery bypass surgery. (Located in the lower leg, the saphenous vein often furnishes short sections that can be used to bypass such blockages.) The research team then isolated from these veins samples of smooth muscle cells (from the vein walls) and endothelial cells (from the vein inner lining). Next, they set about growing these two types of cells in two separate tissue cultures.

To create the new veins, the researchers first rolled up a microscopically thin sheet of biodegradable polymer scaffolding to form a tube. They then harvested the smooth muscle cells, coated the tube with them, and placed the tube in a bioreactor. Approximating the conditions under which blood vessels grow organically in the human body, the bioreactor pulsed a solution of vitamins and nutrients through and around the tube.

Once the smooth muscle cells had proliferated enough to fill the spaces within the scaffold, the researchers added the endothelial cells; this completed the synthetic vein. Finally, the blood vessels were allowed to grow for an additional seven weeks.

Although the finished veins resembled natural blood vessels, they were not strong enough to be implanted in test patients. The Duke researchers see two possible ways to vault this roadblock: They may add different nutrients to the bioreactor, or they may genetically engineer the seed cells to produce more collagen—the protein that lends blood vessels their distinctive structure and strength.

The ability to synthesize blood vessels would be of undeniable benefit to those who require them for heart-bypass surgery. Not only that, but such synthetic channels could help the estimated 100,000 Americans who need small-vessel grafts but cannot get them because their own or prosthetic vessels are unsuitable.

The Stem-Cell Promise

One area of especially cutting-edge cardiology research focuses on growing stem cells into new tissue that can replace damaged or diseased heart muscle. (Stem cells are small populations of unspecialized cells that have the potential to develop into many different types of cells.) Medical teams worldwide are trying to use this technique to repair hearts in one of two ways: by injecting stem cells into the body, or by stimulating the multiplication of stem cells already present.

Human bone marrow, for one, is a rich source of stem cells. Some evidence suggests that stem cells may also reside in the heart—ready to begin producing new heart-muscle cells once they are exposed to the right growth factors or signals.

Dozens of animal experiments have shown that stem cells can be safely introduced into the heart—where, ideally, they take up residence and grow into healthy heart muscle. Several hundred heart patients have likewise participated in stem-cell studies, many of which entailed injecting the cells directly into the heart or introducing them into the bloodstream.

Another approach involves growth factors—hormones or other substances that are infused into the blood or injected directly into damaged heart muscle. The goal here is to stimulate dormant stem cells in the heart to divide and grow into healthy tissue.

So far, these efforts to make stem cells create healthy new heart tissue have met only limited success. Stem-cell studies have not yet achieved major heart-function improvements in patients with heart failure, for example. Nor is there any evidence that stem-cell therapy can prolong the lives of heart-failure patients.

Nonetheless, patients in several small clinical trials seem to have benefited. One such study was described at the American College of Cardiology's 2006 scientific session. Researchers from the University of Hong Kong presented results from the first randomized, placebo-controlled trial to evaluate the effects of injecting bone-marrow cells directly into heart muscle that had been starved of blood and oxygen.

The 28 patients who took part in the study all had advanced coronary artery disease and severe chest pain. None of them had other treatment options. After receiving stem-cell therapy, the patients showed significant improvement both in their exercise capacity and in their hearts' ability to effectively pump blood.

"The heart disease in these patients follows an inexorable downhill course, with disabling symptoms and progressive cardiac failure," said Hung-Fat Tse, M.D., coauthor of the study and deputy director of the Research Center of Heart, Brain, Hormone and Healthy Aging at the University of Hong Kong.

To test the effectiveness of direct injection of bone-marrow cells, Dr. Tse and his colleagues removed bone-marrow cells from the patients with severe CAD and randomly assigned them to receive low- or high-dose injections of bone-marrow cells directly into oxygen-deprived areas of the heart. (Injection allows the maximum number of bone-marrow stem cells to enter the heart muscle.) The control group, meanwhile, received injections of saline solution, a placebo.

After six months, the patients treated with bone-marrow cells were able to exercise for more than one minute, on average, on a treadmill. They also showed a 4 percent increase in the amount of blood pumped out of the left ventricle. Patients receiving the bone-marrow cells also experienced improved ability to perform daily activities and saw reductions in the severity and frequency of their chest pain. The control group, by contrast, showed no improvement in any of these measures.

"Grafting healthy cells into the diseased heart holds enormous potential to induce new blood vessels and strengthen weakened hearts in patients with coronary heart disease," Dr. Tse concluded.

A Scaffold for Heart Repair?

Synthetic versions of biopolymers—large molecules produced by living organisms—are emerging as a promising way to repair damaged hearts. When injected into damaged heart tissue, a biopolymer forms a sort of sticky scaffolding. The cells responsible for repairing and rebuilding heart tissue can then cling to the scaffold as they work, multiplying until they reach cellular levels large enough to reverse or repair the tissue damage.

Biopolymers may prove especially useful when combined with stem-cell therapy designed to heal a damaged heart. The biopolymer fibrin glue contains special chemical-bonding sites; it may thus overcome a historic hurdle to using stem-cell therapy for heart repair: the reluctance of stem cells to stay in place. Stem cells may be able to glom onto these loci, then remain in position long enough to regenerate heart tissue.

New Insight into an Old Drug

When the Greek physician Hippocrates used a powder extracted from willow bark to ease pain and reduce fever in the fifth century B.C., he could scarcely have suspected that he was trailblazing the use of one of the most highly prized drugs in the tattered pageant of pharmaceutical history. The bark of the willow tree contains salicin, a water-soluble crystal that is the key component of acetylsalicylic acid (the active ingredient of aspirin). Today aspirin has been formally marketed in the United States for more than 100 years. (Successfully marketed, too: Americans now pop some 30 billion aspirin tablets a year.)

Many people take aspirin for its coronary benefits—principally its proven ability to forestall a first heart attack or stroke by curbing the tendency of blood to clot. As is the case with any other medication, however, you should never start or stop an aspirin regimen until you have discussed the drug's use with your health care provider.

Medical researchers have recently made additional discoveries about the action and efficacy of aspirin. Among their results were these three key findings:

Aspirin may work better at night. If you use aspirin daily, you may want to give it a nocturnal tweak: Taking aspirin before you go to bed may lower your blood pressure even as the drug performs its main cardiac guard duty of preventing heart attacks and strokes. A small Spanish study found that low-dose aspirin, when taken at night, lowered daytime systolic blood pressure (the top blood-pressure number) by seven points and diastolic pressure (the bottom number) by five points among people who had been newly diagnosed with mild hypertension. Other studies have shown that aspirin appears to be easier on the stomach when swallowed at night.

Aspirin confers different benefits for different sexes. Men and women who take aspirin daily to prevent heart attacks obtain sharply different benefits from doing so.

After reviewing the results of six aspirin studies involving more than 95,000 people, researchers reported in a 2006 *Journal of the American Medical Association* article that aspirin reduces the incidence of strokes in women but not in men. When it comes to heart attacks, by contrast, the reverse holds true: Daily aspirin use reduces the incidence of heart attacks in men but not in women.

Specifically, aspirin treatment lowered the incidence of heart attacks in men by 32 percent but had no effect on their incidence of stroke. For women, aspirin decreased their incidence of stroke by 17 percent but did not significantly mitigate their risk for heart attack.

Both genders share increased odds of one crucial aspirin risk, however: For men as well as women, aspirin use increases the risk of a major bleeding episode by about 70 percent.

Aspirin can help postmenopausal women handle heart disease. For millions of older women who have been diagnosed with heart disease, taking aspirin regularly may constitute a lifesaving therapy.

In findings presented at the annual meeting of the American Heart Association in November 2005, researchers reported their data analysis of more than 90,000 women, ages 50 to 79, who had taken part in the federally funded Women's Health Initiative. The researchers focused on the nearly 10,000 women with cardiovascular disease—including those who had already had a heart attack, stroke, mini-stroke, or cardiac chest pain, or had undergone a procedure such as angioplasty to open clogged coronary arteries.

Taking aspirin regularly, they discovered, significantly reduces the risk of death for older women with heart disease. During more than six years of follow-up, postmenopausal women who regularly took aspirin ran a 17 percent lower risk of dying from any cause than did women who avoided aspirin. These results were identical regardless of the daily aspirin dose, which ranged from 80 milligrams (baby aspirin) to 325 milligrams (the amount in a standard aspirin tablet for adults).

Bloody Important to Know

Warning: For healthy people 70 and over, the risk of serious side effects from aspirin may outweigh the drug's benefits in preventing heart attack and stroke.

In an Australian study, researchers used a computer model to predict what would happen if 20,000 healthy men and women ages 70 to 74 began taking a daily low-dose aspirin. The model was programmed to follow each person until death or age 100. The computer projected that daily aspirin therapy would ward off 765 heart attacks and clot-caused strokes among the sample population. But the predicted aspirin use also precipitated 1,201 cases of major gastrointestinal bleeding and hemorrhagic strokes. The results, by Mark Nelson and colleagues, appeared in the *British Medical Journal* on June 4, 2005.

People of any age can experience side effects from aspirin, but the likelihood of aspirin-associated problems is greater for older people. Aspirin is known to irritate the stomach and gastrointestinal tract, with consequences that transcend mere irritation: Ulceration, gastritis (inflammation of the gastrointestinal tract), and major gastrointestinal bleeding episodes that can cause death.

The findings from this study make it imperative that people over 70 who have not been diagnosed with heart disease but take a daily aspirin for heart health talk to their doctor at once about the wisdom of continuing the therapy.

Indeed, the sole cause for despair among the study results was the fact that a mere 46 percent of the women in the sample had been taking aspirin consistently. According to the study's first author, Duke University cardiology fellow Jeffrey Berger, M.D., there is but one reason that a postmenopausal woman with heart disease should *not* take aspirin: If she is allergic to it or has suffered severe side effects from its use.

Appendices

Resources

American Council on Exercise (ACE)
4851 Paramount Drive
San Diego, California 92123
800-825-3636
www.acefitness.org
This nonprofit organization promotes fitness and a healthy lifestyle. ACE offers a wide variety of educational materials on fitness and provides consumers with information on how to find and evaluate a physical trainer.

American Dietetic Association
120 South Riverside Plaza, Suite 2000
Chicago, Illinois 60606
800-877-1600
www.eatright.org
The association's website offers extensive news and information about nutrition. Call for a referral to a dietitian in your area.

American Heart Association (AHA)
7272 Greenville Avenue
Dallas, Texas 75231
Phone: 800-242-8721
www.americanheart.org
A nonprofit organization, the AHA offers pamphlets and booklets on heart disease and stroke for free or for a nominal fee. Consumers can also call a hotline for answers to questions about heart disease.

Heart Failure Society of America

Court International Suite
240 South, 2550 University Avenue West
St. Paul, Minnesota 55114
651-642-1633
www.hfsa.org
www.abouthf.org

For factual, accurate information about heart failure, this website is among the best. The HFSA—a nonprofit organization made up of specialists in heart-failure care—provides information about heart failure to patients and their families. All of its materials are written and edited by clinical experts.

American Running Association

4405 East West Highway, Suite 405
Bethesda, Maryland 20814
800-776-2732
www.americanrunning.org

This nonprofit organization was founded by doctors to provide runners with resources on training, preventing injury, and reaching fitness goals. The association offers articles on fitness, educational materials, running programs, medical referrals, and listings of races and running clubs. There's even a running-shoe database to help consumers find the proper athletic shoe.

American Society of Hypertension

148 Madison Avenue, 5th Floor
New York, New York 10016
212-696-9099
www.ash-us.org

Contact this organization to find the names of hypertension experts in your area. The society's website offers educational information about high blood pressure, as well as links to other hypertension organizations.

International Society on Hypertension in Blacks, Inc.

2045 Manchester Street NE
Atlanta, Georgia 30324
404-875-6263
www.ishib.org

This organization originally focused on high blood pressure in African Americans but now offers information (including free brochures) on preventing, recognizing, and treating many types of cardiovascular disease, especially in ethnic populations.

National Cholesterol Education Program (NCEP)

NHLBI Health Information Network

P.O. Box 30105

Bethesda, Maryland 20824

301-592-8573

800-575-9355 (consumer hotline with recorded messages)

www.nhlbi.nih.gov

This program of the National Heart, Lung, and Blood Institute maintains a website where members of the public can familiarize themselves with the NCEP guidelines for cholesterol detection and treatment.

National Heart, Lung, and Blood Institute (NHLBI)
Information Center

P.O. Box 30105

Bethesda, Maryland 20824

301-592-8573

www.nhlbi.nih.gov

This division of the National Institutes of Health (NIH) has a website that offers information on many types of heart disease, on diet and exercise, and on the latest Joint National Committee (JNC) guidelines for the prevention, detection, evaluation, and treatment of high blood pressure.

National Hypertension Organization

324 E. 30th Street

New York, New York 1006

212-889-3557

www.nathypertension.org

Use the contact info above to order publications on hypertension, nutrition, and healthy lifestyles.

Weight-control Information Network (WIN)

1 WIN Way

Bethesda, MMaryland 20892-3665

202-828-1025

www.niddk.nih.gov/health/nutrit/win.htm

The National Institute of Diabetes and Digestive and Kidney Diseases joined forces with the National Institutes of Health to create WIN as an information service in 1994. Today, WIN produces and distributes materials on obesity, weight control, and nutrition.

APPENDIX B
Additional Resources from AARP

Personal Medication Record (D18358)
Registro de Medicación (D18396)
The best way to track medications and help the doctor, pharmacist, or other health care professional is to keep a medications list, or Personal Medication Record (PMR). This will help you catalogue the medicines you take (including prescription and over-the-counter drugs and dietary supplements) as well as their dosage amounts and how they are taken.

Medicines Made Easy (D18366)
Medicamentos En Lenguaje Facil (D18511)
This guide shows you how to manage your medications safely and effectively. You'll learn the right questions to ask your health care professionals; the importance of tracking medications; and how to compare drugs for their effectiveness, safety, and price. The guide also includes a Personal Medication Record to complete and share during doctor and pharmacy visits.

The AARP Guide to Pills
www.aarpmagazine.org/books/books_pills.html
This book contains essential information on more than 1,200 life-saving and life-improving prescription and nonprescription medications, including generics. The guide also details side effects and drug interactions. Drugs are listed alphabetically by generic name, then cited by their equivalent brand name. They are conveniently cross-referenced in the index as well.

Physical Activities Workbook (D561)
Too busy to exercise? This workbook shows you how to add physical activity to your daily routine without disrupting your schedule or lifestyle. Learn how to get motivated, start safely, and set goals that meet your health and fitness needs. Also covered: How to develop a personal support network and overcome roadblocks.

The Pocket Guide to Staying Healthy at 50+ (D18010)
La guía para mantenerse saludable después de los 50 (D18024)
This handy guide offers tips and expert advice on good health habits, screening tests, and immunizations. It was developed jointly by AARP and the Agency for Healthcare Research and Quality.

AARP Website: www.aarpmagazine.org/health

APPENDIX C
Dealing with Emergencies

Heart Attack: How Should You Respond?

Knowing the warning signs of a heart attack, and knowing how to respond, could save a life. Because heart attacks may mimic less-serious health conditions such as heartburn, it's important to know the difference between a heart attack and the conditions that resemble it.

The guidelines below can help you make the right decisions and take the right steps when every second counts.

Simple Causes of Chest Pain

Any of the following conditions may cause chest pain:

- Indigestion usually is accompanied by burping, belching, heartburn, nausea, and a sour taste in the mouth.
- A panic attack typically is accompanied by heart palpitations, shortness of breath, and anxiety.
- Chest-wall or muscle pain from exercise or an injury can be made worse by pressing the sore area with a finger.
- The breathing pain of a respiratory infection can often be made worse by coughing or deep breathing.

It is important to know that any of these symptoms can also be present with a heart attack. Do not assume that you are just having indigestion or a panic attack. Get medical help right away.

Heart-Attack Symptoms

You may be having a heart attack or an episode of angina (pain caused when not enough blood reaches the heart muscle) if you have one or more of the following symptoms for no obvious reason:

- Chest pain or constriction, like that of a belt squeezing the chest
- Heaviness in the chest area, as if a heavy weight is resting on the chest
- Pain or pressure in your chest, back, neck, jaw, or arm
- Shortness of breath or trouble breathing
- Pale or gray skin tone and sweating; cool, damp skin
- Nausea or vomiting
- Symptoms that are not relieved by heart medication
- Heavy sweating
- Severe indigestion or heartburn
- Heart palpitations (rapid heartbeat)

Recognizing Silent Problems

Normally, your body warns you of a problem by making you feel pain. But over time, high blood sugar can damage nerves in your body, keeping you from feeling the pain caused by a heart problem. A heart attack with little or no pain is called a silent heart attack. Angina that you're unable to feel is called silent ischemia. Women and people with diabetes have a higher risk for silent heart problems. (NOTE: There may be no pain at all during a silent heart problem.)

Be Prepared

Take the following emergency actions ahead of time if you or a family member has a heart condition or is at risk of a heart attack:

- Know which hospitals in your area provide 24-hour emergency cardiac care. Tell family and friends where these facilities are.
- Post emergency rescue numbers on all of your phones.
- Advise family members and friends to call for emergency care if your chest pain lasts more than a few minutes.

What to Do

1. Call 911 <u>Now!</u>

- Call 911 for emergency medical services. Immediate medical care may keep the heart from stopping and may help minimize damage to the heart muscle.
- Tell the dispatcher where you are and that someone is having a heart attack.
- Don't hang up until told to do so.

2. Keep the Victim Calm

- Persuade the victim to stop all activities.
- Reassure the victim to keep him or her calm. This helps the heart use less oxygen.
- Loosen any clothing that may restrict breathing, such as a tie, a collar, or a belt.

3. Monitor the Victim

- Perform CPR if necessary (see facing page).

4. Wait for Emergency Help to Arrive

- Help the victim get into a relaxed sitting position, with the legs up and bent at the knees. This eases strain on the heart.
- If the victim is conscious and able to swallow, give him or her an adult aspirin with water.
- Remain calm and reassuring.

First Aid: CPR

Cardiopulmonary resuscitation (CPR) is used when the victim is not breathing and has no pulse. CPR combines artificial respiration (which supplies oxygen to the lungs) with chest compression (which circulates oxygen to the brain and other vital organs by forcing blood out of the heart). A CPR class will teach you the correct way to replicate the heart's pumping action. The information below gives you CPR basics only. It is not intended to replace professional instruction.

Before beginning CPR, check to see if the victim is in fact unconscious. Call out to the person, and tap or gently shake him or her. If the person is not conscious, call (or have someone else call) 911 or your local emergency number; that way emergency medical technicians will arrive while you are performing CPR. Then return to the victim and begin CPR.

The ABCs of CPR: Airway, Breathing, Circulation

In order for CPR to be effective, the victim should be lying on his or her back on a flat surface. Kneel down next to the person's neck and shoulders.

Airway

Open the airway by tilting back the head and raising the chin. Listen for breathing.

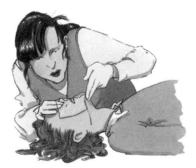

Breathing

If breathing has stopped, pinch the nose, cover the mouth with yours, and blow two full "rescue breaths" into the victim's mouth. Each breath should last about one second

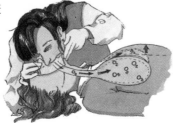

Circulation

Begin chest compressions if the victim is still not breathing normally, coughing, or moving. With your arms straight and parallel to each other, interlace your fingers and position your hands in the center of the chest, between the nipples. Using your upper body weight (not just your arms), push down hard and fast so that you compress the chest by 1-1/2 to 2 inches at a rate of 100 compressions per minute—about two compressions per second. (A CPR course will teach you how to compress the chest correctly. If you perform chest compressions incorrectly, you may injure the victim's ribs or lungs.)

After 30 compressions, open the airway as you did before and give two more rescue breaths lasting one one second each. Provide two rescue breaths and then 30 chest compressions until the person shows signs of consciousness or until help arrives.

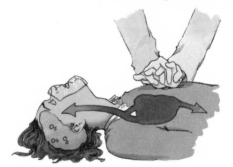

Automated External Defibrillators (AEDs) to Combat Cardiac Arrest

More than 200,000 Americans die of sudden cardiac arrest each year, says the American Red Cross. Cases of sudden cardiac arrest usually result from abnormal heart rhythms (arrhythmias). The large majority of cases are due to ventricular fibrillation—a condition in which the heart's electrical impulses suddenly become so chaotic that the heart can no longer pump blood effectively. (Chapter 6 explains ventricular fibrillation in greater detail.)

What triggers the arrhythmias that cause sudden cardiac arrest? Medical researchers aren't sure. Many victims have no history of heart disease. And unlike the majority of people who experience heart attacks, many victims of sudden cardiac arrest have had no prior warning symptoms.

Victims of sudden cardiac arrest collapse and quickly lose consciousness. The heart has essentially stopped beating, so death will occur in a matter of minutes unless a normal heart rhythm can be restored.

Fortunately, small, portable devices called automated external defibrillators (AEDs) have the potential to keep a person from dying of sudden cardiac arrest. Indeed, AEDs have become nearly as prevalent as wall-mounted fire extinguishers. You've probably spotted them in their characteristic laptop-sized boxes on walls or pillars in corporate offices, airports, shopping malls, sports stadiums, schools, community centers, and other places where people congregate. Typically, these containers are placed below signs featuring a red heart with a bolt of lightning in the middle of it. To see a sample of the AED sign, visit www.aedsuperstore.com and click on "AED Walls Signs and Decals."

How to Use an AED

An AED is simple to use. It emits voice prompts to instruct the rescuer. In just a few seconds, the AED analyzes a person's heart rhythm for abnormalities. Based on what it finds, it may then instruct the rescuer to deliver an electrical shock to the victim's heart. This shock, known as defibrillation, jolts the heart into resuming a more normal rhythm.

The chance of surviving sudden cardiac arrest decreases by 10 percent for each minute that a person's heart is not beating. For this reason, rapid defibrillation through the use of an AED offers the greatest hope for surviving cardiac arrest.

What Should You Do?

A person in cardiac arrest lies motionless, without breathing. He or she will not respond to questions, shaking, or other stimulation. On encountering someone who appears to be in this condition, find out whether the person is conscious by asking loudly, "Are you okay?"

If there is no response, turn the person on his or her back. Then look, listen, and feel to find out whether breathing has stopped:

- **Look** to see whether the chest is moving up and down;
- **Listen** for sounds of breathing;
- **Feel** for air movement above the person's mouth.

If breathing cannot be detected, look inside the mouth and throat and remove any objects that may be blocking the airway. Then, if an AED is available, use it immediately as first aid for cardiac arrest.

When the AED is turned on, you will be prompted to apply to the victim's chest the two paddles (electrode patches) that come with the AED. Once these are applied, the AED will monitor the victim's heart rhythm. If the device detects a "shockable" rhythm, it will charge itself up, then instruct you to stand clear of the victim and press the shock button.

After the AED has discharged its electrical shock, call for professional medical assistance. If the person has not resumed breathing, begin CPR (see CPR instructions, page TK).

The American Red Cross and the American Heart Association offer training in CPR and in the use of AEDs. For information on the time and location of training classes, contact your local chapter of either organization.

Index

benefits of, 42–43, 88–89, 104, 139, 141, 147, 149, 169, 232
blood pressure and, 141, 142
for cardiac rehab, 221–229
cholesterol levels and, 46, 47, 147, 149, 169
cooling down after, 94
diabetes and, 51, 91, 229–230
easing into, 90–93
fitness for life, 105–106
habits, 92, 228
increasing activity generally and, 92
log, 103–104
measuring exertion, 93–95, 223–227
organizations, 251, 252
overcoming obstacles to, 88
overexertion signs, 199, 226
overweight/weight loss and, 52, 132
questions about, 89
rewards for, 104–105
right kind of, 92
safety and comfort, 90
before starting, 89
stem-cell therapy affecting, 245, 246
strength exercises, 101–103, 223
stress and, 139, 221–223, 232
stretching before/after, 94, 95–100, 223
taking pulse during, 95, 224–225
talk test during, 94, 223
walking, 92–93, 198, 223–224
warming up before, 94
warning signs during/after, 96, 199
Exercise test (stress ECG), 77–79, 204, 222
Ezetimibe (Zetia®), 168

Fainting (syncope), 17, 22, 27, 64–67, 194, 204, 209
Fatigue, 15, 62, 71–72, 73, 79, 226
Fats, 112–116, 121, 122, 134–135, 147–148. See also Cholesterol; High-density lipoprotein (HDL); Low-density lipoprotein (LDL)
Fibrates, 168
First Aid. See Emergency responses
Fitness. See Exercise; Physical activity
Fluttering feeling, 27, 68, 204, 210. See also Atrial fibrillation; Atrial flutter

Food. See Diet
Food labels
foods without, 116
reading, 112–114, 118, 133–135, 144–145, 197

Gene therapy, 239, 241

Hamstring stretch, 100
Head tilt, 96
Health history, 73
Health, tracking, 203
Heart
chambers, 2–3
illustrated, 4, 5, 6
interior structure of, 2–3
main functions of, 2
mechanical functioning of, 1–2, 3–9
as muscle, 1–3
Heart attack
artery blockage causing, 63
causes of, 174
chest pain indicating, 61
defined, 13
symptoms, 175, 257
Heart attack treatment, 174–190
angioplasty, 175–176, 177–181
bypass grafting (CABG). See also Coronary artery bypass graft (CABG) surgery
clot-dissolving drugs, 61, 174–175
emergency angioplasty, 174–176
finding blocked arteries, 176–177
immediate response, 174
stenting, 181–183, 238
Heart beat
amount per day/lifetime, 2
mechanics of, 5–6
taking pulse, 95, 224–225
Heart disease, 11–31. See also specific diseases
deaths from, xiii
knowledge benefits, xiv–xv
overview, 11
statistics, xiii–xiv
Heart failure, 17–18
ACE inhibitors for, 199
activity and, 198
alcohol and, 169

taking blood pressure, 41–42
treating/controlling, 35, 42–44,
141–147, 156–164, 241–242

ICD (implantable cardioverter
defibrillator), 209–212
Implantable cardioverter defibrillator
(ICD), 209–212
International Society of Hypertension
in Blacks, Inc, 253
Intimacy and sex, after heart disease,
230–234

LDL. *See* Low-density lipoprotein
(LDL)
Lifestyle changes
for cholesterol, 147–149
for hypertension, 140–147
Limb pain or failure. *See* Claudication;
Peripheral arterial disease (PAD)
Low-density lipoprotein (LDL), 34. *See
also* Cholesterol
characteristics of, 36, 46
controlling, 46–48
HDL vs., 36, 45, 46
high, causes of, 37, 112, 113,
114–115, 135
levels, 45, 46, 56, 165
lowering, 126, 135, 147–149,
165–170, 238
metabolic syndrome and, 49–50

Medications
for angina, 172–174
chart, 153
educating yourself/others about,
151–154
for heart failure, 198–200
for heart-failure-related conditions,
200
for heart-valve disease, 213–214
for high cholesterol, 165–169
for hypertension, 157–164
intravenous (IV), 200
for raising HDL, 239–240
routine for, 201
side effects, 200. See also specific
medications
taking, 201

tracking, 153, 201
Medications (specific types)
ACE inhibitors, 161–163, 199, 214
aliskiren (Razilez®), 241–242
antibiotics, 214
anticoagulants, 200, 205–207, 214,
215, 247–249
ARBs, 163
beta blockers, 160–161, 199, 214
calcium-channel blockers, 163
chemical cardioversion, 205
clot-dissolving drugs, 174–175
digitalis medicines, 200, 213–214
diuretics, 158–159, 200, 213
experimental blocker, 239–240
ezetimibe (Zetia®), 168
fibrates, 168
hydralazine, 199
Milano protein, 239
niacin, 168–169
nitrates, 199
nitroglycerin, 172–174
orlistat (Xenical®), 240
rimonabant (Acomplia®), 240
sibutramine (Meridia®), 240
statins, 165–167, 239–240
thrombolytic drugs, 174–175
torcetrapib, 239–240
warfarin, 205–207
Meridia® (sibutramine), 240
Metabolic syndrome, 36, 49–50
Milano protein, 239
Mitral insufficiency, 26
Mitral stenosis, 26–27
Mitral valve, 6, 22, 23, 237
Mitral-valve prolapse, 25–26
MUGA scan, 76
Myocardium, 3, 61

National Cholesterol Education
Program (NCEP), 253
National Heart, Lung, and Blood
Institute (NHLBI), 253
National Hypertension Organization,
253
Niacin, 168–169
Nitrates, 199
Nitroglycerin, 172–174
Nuclear testing, cardiac, 75–77

causing chest pain, 257
diuretics and, 158
exercise and, 89, 198
during exercise test, 79
fluid in lungs and, 19
heart attacks and, 61, 175, 257
heart failure and, 18, 191, 193, 197
heart-valve disease and, 22
palpitations and, 69
prescription drugs and, 213
during sex, 233
when to call doctor, 85, 89, 96, 175,
183, 191
Shoulder press, 102
Shoulder roll, 97
Sibutramine (Meridia®), 240
Silent killer. See Hypertension (high
blood pressure)
Silent problems, recognizing, 258
Sinoatrial (SA) node, 3, 5, 6
Smoking, 48–49, 125–130
benefits of quitting, 126
blood pressure and, 43
gauging risks from, 48
lowering risk from, 49
new treatment for, 240
quitting, 127–130, 131, 240
rating risk of, 126–127
risks, 35, 48, 125–126
Sodium (salt) intake, 116–117, 118,
121, 142–147
Statins, 165–167, 239–240
Stem-cell research, 244–246
Stenting, 181–183, 238
Strength exercises, 101–103, 223
Stress, 137–140
angina and, 15
blood pressure and, 44
dangers of, 53–55
defined, 137
exercise and, 139, 221–223, 232
fatigue and, 71–72
hypertension and, 156
preventing/reducing, 37, 44,
129–130, 139–140, 141, 220–221,
223, 231
relaxation techniques, 129–130,
139
responding to, 137–138, 217

risks, 34, 36
targeting triggers, 54
Stress test. See Exercise test (stress
ECG)
Stretching muscles, 94, 95–100, 223
Stroke
heeding signs of, 31
risk of, 28–30
symptoms, 30–31
Surgery. See also Coronary artery
bypass graft (CABG) surgery
for heart-valve disease, 24, 25, 26,
202, 214–215, 236–237, 267
rebuilding intimacy after, 230–234
rehab after. See Cardiac rehab;
Recovering, from heart disease
Swelling. See Edema (swelling)
Symptoms. See also Edema (swelling);
Shortness of breath (dyspnea)
alerting doctor about, 59–60
of atrial fibrillation, 27
as changes in body, 59
charting, 203
chest pain, 60–64. See also Angina
claudication (limb pain or fatigue),
69–71
defined, 59
fainting (syncope), 17, 22, 27,
64–67, 194, 204, 209
fatigue, 15, 62, 71–72, 73, 79, 226
of heart attacks, 175, 257
of heart failure, 18, 71–72, 190–191,
209
of heart-valve disease, 22
heeding, 73
palpitations, 15, 25, 27, 62, 67–69,
73, 204, 257
of strokes, 30–31
Syncope (fainting), 17, 22, 27, 64–67,
194, 204, 209
Synthetic biopolymers, 246–247
Synthetic blood vessels, 243–244
Systolic dysfunction, 18, 191, 192

Tests
calcium scan, 84–85
cardiac catheterization, 79–81
cardiac nuclear testing, 75–77
echocardiogram, 74–75